Emergent Pulmonary Embolism Management in Hospital Practice

From Hyperacute to Follow-Up Care

Emergent Pulmonary Embolism Management in Hospital Practice

From Hyperacute to Follow-Up Care

Editors

Colm McCabe
Royal Brompton Hospital, UK

Aaron Waxman
Brigham and Women's Hospital, USA

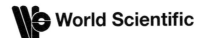 **World Scientific**

NEW JERSEY · LONDON · SINGAPORE · BEIJING · SHANGHAI · HONG KONG · TAIPEI · CHENNAI · TOKYO

Published by

World Scientific Publishing Europe Ltd.

57 Shelton Street, Covent Garden, London WC2H 9HE

Head office: 5 Toh Tuck Link, Singapore 596224

USA office: 27 Warren Street, Suite 401-402, Hackensack, NJ 07601

Library of Congress Cataloging-in-Publication Data
Names: McCabe, Colm, editor. | Waxman, Aaron B., editor.
Title: Emergent pulmonary embolism management in hospital practice : from hyperacute
    to follow-up care / editors, Colm McCabe, Royal Brompton Hospital, UK,
    Aaron Waxman, Brigham and Women's Hospital, USA.
Description: Hackensack, New Jersey : World Scientific, [2023] |
    Includes bibliographical references and index.
Identifiers: LCCN 2022025585 | ISBN 9781800612761 (hardcover) |
    ISBN 9781800612778 (ebook for institutions) | ISBN 9781800612785 (ebook for individuals)
Subjects: MESH: Pulmonary Embolism--therapy | Emergency Service, Hospital |
    Emergency Medical Services--methods
Classification: LCC RC694.3 | NLM WG 420 | DDC 616.1/35025--dc23/eng/20220727
LC record available at https://lccn.loc.gov/2022025585

British Library Cataloguing-in-Publication Data
A catalogue record for this book is available from the British Library.

For any available supplementary material, please visit
https://www.worldscientific.com/worldscibooks/10.1142/Q0376#t=suppl

Desk Editors: Balasubramanian Shanmugam/Adam Binnie/Shi Ying Koe

Typeset by Stallion Press
Email: enquiries@stallionpress.com

Preface

Acute pulmonary embolism is a condition which, more than most, has benefitted from a wealth of evidence that justifies diagnostic and treatment approaches, both contemporary and historical. Treatment strategies in pulmonary embolism have also been recently incorporated into highly developed European guidelines which, to the interested reader, provide definitive practice recommendations. One may ask therefore the purpose of a textbook that addresses several aspects of its diagnosis and management given the wealth of recent resource?

Put simply, the aim of this book is to address gaps in evidence and provide practical descriptions and advice to clinicians treating pulmonary embolism where management decisions may not be immediately straightforward. While not all suggestions may be backed by wealth of evidence, pulmonary embolism has seen an explosion in the application of new technologies, both pharmacological and interventional, within the acute care setting many of which are currently insufficiently studied (or understood) to qualify for guideline inclusion. Notwithstanding this evidence gap, clinicians must also continue to deliver the best possible care in an increasingly complex patient cohort with very specific management dilemmas.

In compiling contributions for this book, we have attempted as far as possible to include in narrative form suggested approaches to pulmonary embolism treatment from contributors with extensive first-hand experience of each aspect and so offer something extra to both experienced and more junior clinicians, general and specialist, beyond what may be gleaned from current guidelines. We hope this book will be helpful in day to day clinical practice, and that the reader will be enthused to delve deeper into areas of specific interest or uncertainty.

About the Editors

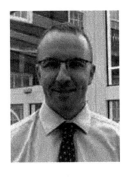

Colm McCabe is a consultant respiratory physician and lead for exercise services in Cardiology at the Royal Brompton Hospital, as well as holding an Honorary Senior Lecturer position at Imperial College, London. His training includes a research MD at Papworth Hospital, Cambridge; a clinical fellowship in exercise physiology funded by the award of the Scadding Morriston Davies and Berkeley Fellowships (UCL with Gonville and Caius); and a Masters from the University of Bologna. His clinical interest lies in all forms of pulmonary vascular disease and he is currently engaged in several translation research projects related to acute and chronic pulmonary embolism, holding several research grants in this field.

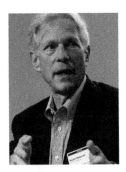

Aaron Waxman, MD, PhD, is the Executive Director of the Center for Pulmonary Heart Diseases at the Brigham and Women's Hospital, and works in the Heart and Vascular, and Lung Centers. He is an Associate Professor of Medicine at Harvard Medical School with appointments in the Division of Pulmonary Critical Care Medicine and Cardiovascular Medicine. His interests have focused on developing a translational centre that integrates clinical and basic research and focuses on a better understanding of the pathogenesis of pulmonary vascular remodelling and the physiology of right ventricular adaptation to changes in the pulmonary vascular bed. His academic concentrations include the role of inflammatory mediators in pulmonary vascular remodelling and right ventricular–pulmonary arterial coupling.

List of Contributors

Deepa J. Arachchillage, MD, MRCP, FRCPath, Department of Haematology, Imperial College Healthcare NHS Trust, London, UK (deepa.jayakodyarachchillage@nhs.net)

Karen A. Breen, MD, MRCPI, FRCPath, Department of Haematology, Guy's and St Thomas' NHS Foundation Trust, London, UK (Karen.Breen@gstt.nhs.uk)

Andrew Constantine, MBBS, MA, Department of Cardiology, Royal Brompton and Harefield Hospitals, Guy's and St Thomas' NHS Foundation Trust, London, UK (A.Constantine@rbht.nhs.uk)

Christina Crossette-Thambiah, MBBS, BSc, MRCP, Imperial College Healthcare NHS Trust, London, UK (c.crossette-thambiah@nhs.net)

Chris Davies, MD, FRCP, Department of Respiratory Medicine, University Hospitals Dorset NHS Trust, UK (cwhdavies@doctors.org.uk)

Benjamin Garfield, BMBS, PhD, Royal Brompton and Harefield Hospitals, Guy's and St Thomas' NHS Foundation Trust, London, UK (B.Garfield@rbht.nhs.uk)

Elizabeth B. Gay, MD, Assistant Professor of Medicine, Harvard Medical School, Division of Pulmonary Critical Care Medicine, Brigham and Women's Hospital, Harvard Medical School, Boston, MA, USA (egay@bwh.harvard.edu)

Eileen Harder, MD, Burke Fellow in Pulmonary Vascular Disease, Division of Pulmonary Critical Care Medicine, Brigham and Women's Hospital, Harvard Medical School, Boston, MA, USA (eharder1@bwh.harvard.edu)

Luke Howard, DPhil, FRCP, Department of Cardiology, Imperial College Healthcare NHS Trust, UK (l.howard@imperial.ac.uk)

Menno V. Huisman, MD, PhD, Department of Thrombosis and Hemostasis, Leiden University Medical Center, Leiden, the Netherlands (m.v.huisman@lumc.nl)

Narayan Karunanithy, MRCS, FRCR, FCIRSE, School of Biomedical Engineering & Imaging Science, Faculty of Life Science & Medicine, King's College London, London, UK (Narayan.Karunanithy@gstt.nhs.uk)

Aleksander Kempny, MD, PhD, Department of Cardiology, Royal Brompton and Harefield Hospitals, Guy's and St Thomas' NHS Foundation Trust, London, UK (A.Kempny@rbht.nhs.uk)

Akhil Khosla, MD, Section of Pulmonary, Critical Care, and Sleep Medicine, Yale School of Medicine, New Haven, CT, USA (akhil.khosla@yale.edu)

Frederikus A. Klok, MD, PhD, FESC, Department of Thrombosis and Hemostasis, Leiden University Medical Center, Leiden, the Netherlands (F.A.Klok@lumc.nl)

Charlie Lee, MMSc, MPAS, PA-C, Division of Pulmonary Critical Care Medicine, Brigham and Women's Hospital, Harvard Medical School, Boston, MA, USA (clee39@bwh.harvard.edu)

Colm McCabe, MD, Department of Cardiology, Royal Brompton and Harefield Hospitals, Guy's and St Thomas' NHS Foundation Trust, London, UK (c.mccabe2@rbht.nhs.uk)

Bhashkar Mukherjee, MBBChir, PhD, Guy's and St Thomas' NHS Foundation Trust, London, UK (Bhashkar.Mukherjee@gstt.nhs.uk)

Simon Padley, BSc, MBBS, FRCP, FRCR, Department of Radiology, Royal Brompton and Harefield Hospitals, Guy's and St Thomas' NHS Foundation Trust, London, UK (S.Padley@rbht.nhs.uk)

Mariana Pfeferman, BS, Division of Cardiovascular Medicine, Brigham and Women's Hospital, Harvard Medical School, Boston, MA, USA (maripfef@gmail.com)

Gregory Piazza, MD, MS, Associate Professor of Medicine, Harvard Medical School, Division of Cardiovascular Medicine, Brigham and Women's Hospital, Harvard Medical School, Boston, MA, USA (gpiazza@bwh.harvard.edu)

Laura C. Price, PhD, FRCP, Department of Cardiology, Royal Brompton and Harefield Hospitals, Guy's and St Thomas' NHS Foundation Trust, London, UK (Laura.Price@rbht.nhs.uk)

Susanna Price, MD, PhD, Royal Brompton and Harefield Hospitals, Guy's and St Thomas' NHS Foundation Trust, London, UK (S.Price@rbht.nhs.uk)

Carole Ridge, MB, BCh, BAO, MRCPI, FFRRCSI, Department of Radiology, Royal Brompton and Harefield Hospitals, Guy's and St Thomas' NHS Foundation Trust, London, UK (C.Ridge@rbht.nhs.uk)

Wei Qi, MD, Research Fellow in Medicine, Division of Pulmonary Critical Care Medicine, Brigham and Women's Hospital, Harvard Medical School, Boston, MA, USA (wqi2@bwh.harvard.edu)

Chinthaka B. Samaranayake, MBChB, FRACP, Royal Brompton and Harefield Hospitals, Guy's and St Thomas' NHS Foundation Trust, London, UK (C.Samaranayake@rbht.nhs.uk)

Stella M. Savarimuthu, MD, Section of Pulmonary, Critical Care, and Sleep Medicine, Yale School of Medicine, New Haven, CT, USA (stella. savarimuthu@yale.edu)

Karina C. Shuttie, MPAS, PA-C, Division of Pulmonary Critical Care Medicine, Brigham and Women's Hospital, Harvard Medical School, Boston, MA, USA (kshuttie@bwh.harvard.edu)

Inderjit Singh, MD, Assistant Professor of Medicine, Section of Pulmonary, Critical Care, and Sleep Medicine, Yale School of Medicine, New Haven, CT, USA (inderjit.singh@yale.edu)

Milou A.M. Stals, MD, Department of Thrombosis and Hemostasis, Leiden University Medical Center, Leiden, the Netherlands (m.a.m.stals@lumc.nl)

David M. Systrom, MD, Assistant Professor of Medicine, Harvard Medical School, Division of Pulmonary Critical Care Medicine, Brigham and Women's Hospital, Harvard Medical School, Boston, MA, USA (dsystrom@bwh.harvard.edu)

Richard Trimlett, AFICM, FRCS, FRCS(CTh), Royal Brompton and Harefield Hospitals, Guy's and St Thomas' NHS Foundation Trust, London, UK (R.Trimlett@rbht.nhs.uk)

Bavithra Vijayakumar, MBBS, BSc, MRCP, Royal Brompton and Harefield Hospitals, Guy's and St Thomas' NHS Foundation Trust, London, UK (bavithra.vijayakumar@nhs.net)

Aaron B. Waxman, MD, PhD, Associate Professor of Medicine, Harvard Medical School, Division of Pulmonary Critical Care Medicine, Brigham and Women's Hospital, Harvard Medical School, Boston, MA, USA (abwaxman@bwh.harvard.edu)

S. John Wort, PhD, FRCP, Department of Cardiology, Royal Brompton and Harefield Hospitals, Guy's and St Thomas' NHS Foundation Trust, London, UK (S.Wort@rbht.nhs.uk)

Contents

**Chapter 2 Correct Risk Stratification at Diagnosis — Why
It Matters?**   **17**
Mariana Pfeferman and Gregory Piazza

**Chapter 3 Outpatient Management of Pulmonary
Embolism: Who Can I Send Home?**   **29**
Bavithra Vijayakumar and Chris Davies

Part 1

Acute Care

https://doi.org/10.1142/9781800612778_0001

Chapter 1

Getting the Diagnosis of Acute Pulmonary Embolism Right — Which Diagnostic Strategy?

Milou A.M. Stals, Menno V. Huisman, and Frederikus A. Klok

Leiden University Medical Center, Leiden, The Netherlands

Abstract

Various fast and non-invasive diagnostic strategies for ruling out pulmonary embolism have been developed over the last decades, with the aim of simplifying the diagnostic management of patients with suspected pulmonary embolism, and to reduce the number of required imaging tests. These strategies all start with the assessment of pre-test probability using a validated clinical decision rule, and a D-dimer blood test. The combination of a non-high clinical probability and a normal D-dimer test safely rules out PE, while all other patients should be referred for imaging tests, which nowadays mostly concerns computed tomography pulmonary angiography (CTPA). The recent introduction of age- or pre-test-probability-dependent D-dimer thresholds have greatly improved the specificity of the D-dimer test and allow for more patients to be managed without a CTPA. In this chapter, we discuss how these algorithms are largely applicable to relevant patient subgroups such as the elderly, patients with cancer, pregnant women, and patients with COVID-19 pneumonia.

Introduction

Pulmonary embolism (PE), together with deep vein thrombosis (DVT) referred to as venous thromboembolism (VTE), is a leading cause of cardiovascular mortality, and an accurate and timely diagnosis is therefore very important. However, the diagnosis of PE is challenging, even among experienced clinicians, as signs and symptoms of PE are varied and non-specific. The "classic" symptoms of acute PE are acute dyspnoea and (pleuritic) chest pain, but patients can also present with syncope (fainting), palpitations, haemoptysis (coughing up blood), or concurrent symptoms of DVT. On the other hand, PE can also be asymptomatic and only discovered incidentally on imaging tests for another disease. Altogether, signs and symptoms of PE lack diagnostic accuracy and objective imaging tests are required to confirm the diagnosis. Yet, imaging tests are time-consuming, costly, and associated with radiation exposure and contrast material-induced complications. Moreover, as other cardiopulmonary diseases present with overlapping symptoms, the proportion of confirmed PE cases among patients investigated for the disease is low (around 10–20%) and the majority of the patients will not have PE. In fact, this proportion of confirmed PE cases is decreasing steadily over recent decades, as clinicians tend to initiate testing for PE more frequently than in the past. Therefore, various diagnostic strategies for ruling out PE were developed, with the aim of simplifying the diagnostic management of patients with suspected PE, and to reduce the number of required imaging tests.

Diagnostic Strategies

Any diagnostic strategy starts with a clinical suspicion of PE. None of the diagnostic tests discussed later should be used as a screening tool for possible PE in an unselected population of patients with respiratory or chest symptoms. If testing for PE is warranted, recommended diagnostic strategies for ruling out PE consist of assessment of the clinical pre-test probability using validated clinical decision rules (CDRs) and D-dimer testing. The combination of a non-high clinical probability and a normal D-dimer test safely rules out PE, without the need for imaging tests. Of note, these non-invasive diagnostic strategies are to be used in haemodynamically stable patients only. In patients with hemodynamic instability, emergency chest imaging is recommended, may be even with the administration of therapeutic anticoagulants prior to objective diagnosis.

Step 1: Assessment of Clinical Pre-Test Probability

Clinical pre-test probability (CPTP) assessment can be performed either by implicit (empirical) clinical judgement or by using validated standardised CDRs. Several CDRs have been developed in recent decades, of which the most extensively validated and widely used CDRs are the Wells rule and the revised Geneva score. These scores incorporate clinical signs, symptoms, and predisposing factors for VTE, to classify patients with suspected PE into categories of pre-test probability. Ultimately, the goal of CPTP is to (1) select patients with a non-high CPTP in whom PE can be ruled out after a negative D-dimer test and imaging safely withheld and (2) select patients with a high CPTP who do require imaging tests to confirm or rule out the diagnosis of PE, irrespective of D-dimer testing.

The Wells rule and revised Geneva score consist of seven and eight items, respectively (Table 1). Both scores include nearly the same items (e.g., active malignancy, previous VTE, haemoptysis, and clinical signs of DVT) and they assign different weights to these various items. But whereas the Wells rule includes the subjective item "whether PE is assessed as the most likely diagnosis", the revised Geneva score was constructed as an objective CDR and does not include this item. The judgement of this latter item was much criticised in the past, as it is subjective, presumably critically dependent on clinical experience, and carries major weight in the final score. Nonetheless, the reported interobserver variability of the Wells score proved to be good, and it has been shown that assessing the score is independent of the clinician's experience. The original Wells and revised Geneva scores classify patients into three categories of CPTP: low, intermediate and high, whereas the later proposed dichotomised scores classify patients as PE unlikely or PE likely (Table 1). The effectiveness of both the three-level and the two-level scores have been demonstrated extensively.

More recently, the YEARS algorithm was developed. This algorithm consists of only three items from the original Wells score, i.e., clinical signs of DVT, haemoptysis, and whether PE is the most likely diagnosis. Patients are classified in two groups: patient with zero YEARS items and patients with 1–3 YEARS items. In the YEARS algorithm, all patients qualify for D-dimer testing (Table 1).

The accuracy of these different CDRs was evaluated in several meta-analyses. In addition, one formal prospective management study directly compared the Wells rule with the revised Geneva score. These

Table 1.   The Wells rule, revised Geneva score, and the YEARS algorithm.

CDRs	Wells rule		Revised Geneva score		YEARS algorithm	
Items and points	Haemoptysis	1	Age >65y	1	Clinical signs of DVT	1
	Active malignancy	1	Surgery or fracture <1 month	2	Haemoptysis	1
	Prior history of VTE	1.5	Active malignancy	2	PE most likely diagnosis	1
	Surgery or immobilisation <4 weeks	1.5	Haemoptysis	2		
	Heart rate >100 bpm	1.5	Prior history of VTE	3		
	Clinical signs of DVT	3	Unilateral lower limb pain	3		
	PE most likely diagnosis	3	Heart rate	75–94 bpm: 3 ≥95 bpm: 5		
			Pain on lower limb palpation and unilateral edema	4		
Pre-test probability assessment	**Original classification**		**Original classification**		**Original classification**	
	Three-level score		*Three-level score*			
	Low	0–1.5	Low	0–3	Low	0
	Intermediate	2–6	Intermediate	4–10	Moderate/ high	1–3
	High	>6	High	>10		
	Two-level score		*Two-level score*			
	PE unlikely	0–4	PE unlikely	0–5		
	PE likely	>4	PE likely	>5		
	For D-dimer dependent on CPTP		For D-dimer dependent on CPTP			
	Low	0–4	Low	0–5		
	Moderate	4.5–6	Moderate	6–10		
	High	>6	High	>10		

Notes: CDR: clinical decision rule; VTE: venous thromboembolism; bpm: beats per minute; DVT: deep-vein thrombosis; PE: pulmonary embolism; CPTP: clinical pre-test probability assessment; y: years.

studies measure diagnostic performance of the strategies by using the outcomes "safety" and "efficiency". Safety is defined in these studies as the failure rate, which is the 3-month incidence of VTE after excluding PE without imaging at baseline (actually a measure of missed diagnosis at baseline; of which the recommended safety threshold traditionally ranges between 2% and 3%), while efficiency is defined as the number of patients in whom imaging could be avoided. Results of the aforementioned studies showed that the diagnostic performance of the evaluated CDRs was equivalent. Consequently, the choice for a specific CDR depends on local preference and experience, in accordance with current guidelines.

Step 2: D-Dimer Testing

D-dimer testing is the next step in patients with a non-high CPTP, or in all patients in the YEARS algorithm. As D-dimer is a degradation product of cross-linked fibrin, D-dimer levels are typically elevated in patients with VTE. Consequently, D-dimer testing has a high sensitivity and a normal D-dimer level renders a diagnosis of PE unlikely. However, since D-dimer levels are elevated in other common clinical conditions as well (e.g., increased age, malignancy, pregnancy, infection, trauma, and post-operatively), the specificity of D-dimer is low. The strength of D-dimer testing thus lies in ruling out PE.

A large variety of assays are available for D-dimer testing. Most often quantitative enzyme-linked immunosorbent assays (ELISA) or ELISA-derived assays are used, with a high diagnostic sensitivity of 95–99.5%. Although qualitative D-dimer test assays have a lower sensitivity than the quantitative test assays, they are being used in practice, most often as point of care tests in the community.

For the quantitative tests, different D-dimer thresholds exist. Previously, the D-dimer threshold was fixed at 500 μg/L. While this threshold was proven to be safe (i.e., failure rate <1% in patients with non-high CPTP and normal D-dimer test), PE could only be ruled out without imaging in about ~30% of the patients. Efficiency was even lower (about 10–15%) in specific patient populations (e.g., patients with cancer, elderly patients, and patients with history of VTE). In order to improve efficiency of D-dimer testing, age-adjusted D-dimer thresholds and D-dimer thresholds dependent on CPTP were developed.

The age-adjusted D-dimer threshold is calculated as age × 10 μg/L for patients above 50 years of age. When applying this threshold in patients under the age of 50, the fixed D-dimer threshold of 500 μg/L applies. The D-dimer threshold dependent on CPTP applies a higher threshold in patients with a low CPTP (i.e., threshold of 1,000 μg/L in patients with low CPTP, and threshold of 500 μg/L in patients with moderate CPTP). This CPTP dependent D-dimer threshold has been validated in combination with both the YEARS algorithm and the Wells rule. These adapted D-dimer thresholds have increased the proportion of patients in whom PE can safely be ruled out without imaging considerably, with efficiencies of up to 50–60% in the general patient population. Moreover, a further reduction in imaging tests could also be achieved in specific patient populations, with efficiencies of 15–30% in for instance patients with cancer, elderly patients or patients with a history of VTE. Therefore, current guidelines state that these adapted D-dimer thresholds should be considered as an alternative to the fixed D-dimer threshold.

In some specific situations, such as patients with a history suggestive of PE for more than 14 days and patients already receiving therapeutic anticoagulant therapy, D-dimer testing must be used with caution or even be avoided. These patients were often excluded from the available studies, and as a result, little evidence is available on the safety of their use in these patients. Some studies suggest that D-dimer tests may give more false-negative results in these patients.

Imaging Tests

Following the diagnostic strategies, imaging is required in patients with a high CPTP and/or abnormal D-dimer test (Figure 1). In the past, pulmonary angiography (PA) was the gold standard imaging test for diagnosing PE. However, PA is an invasive technique, as it requires right heart catheterisation and injection of contrast material. Nowadays, computed tomographic pulmonary angiography (CTPA) has replaced PA as the first-choice imaging test for suspected PE (example of CTPA images; see Figure 2).

Computed tomographic pulmonary angiography

CTPA is the imaging method of choice in patients with suspected PE. CTPA requires the injection of iodinated contrast material, after which CTPA can be performed within 4–5 seconds. PE is diagnosed in

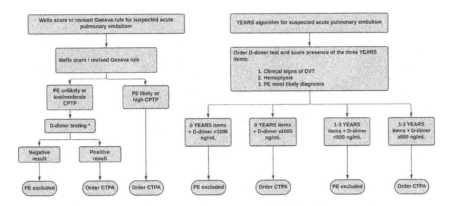

Figure 1. Diagnostic strategies for ruling out PE.

Notes: PE: pulmonary embolism; CPTP: clinical pre-test probability assessment; CTPA: CT pulmonary angiography; DVT: deep vein thrombosis.

*D-dimer testing: fixed (<500 μg/L) or age-adjusted D-dimer testing (<age × 10 μg/L in patients aged >50 years) in PE unlikely patients, or D-dimer testing dependent on CPTP (<1,000 ng/mL for a low clinical probability and <500 ng/mL for a moderate clinical probability) in patients with a low and moderate CPTP, respectively.

Reproduced with permission from Stals *et al.* (2022).

the case of an intraluminal filling defect, which can be visualised down to the subsegmental level. The sensitivity and specificity of CTPA has improved considerably by the introduction of multidetector-row CT scanners (MD-CTPA). With these scanners, a high sensitivity (96–100%) and specificity (97–98%) could be reached. The safety of using MD-CTPA as a stand-alone imaging test has been confirmed by several studies. A negative CTPA result thus adequately excludes the diagnosis of PE.

Despite all these advantages, some pitfalls remain with the use of CTPA as the first-choice imaging method. First of all, as CTPA is easily accessible, clinicians tend to overuse this technique with the risk of over-diagnosing smaller (isolated) subsegmental emboli due to the more sensitive scanning techniques, with unknown clinical relevance. Besides, motion artefacts, which are particularly prevalent in patients suffering from severe dyspnoea, can mimic intraluminal filling defects on CTPA scans, which are consequently misdiagnosed as PE. This overdiagnosing is relevant as well, as it may expose patients to the risk of bleeding complications associated with anticoagulant therapy.

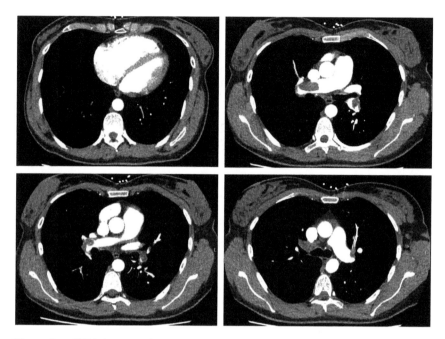

Figure 2. CTPA images of a patient with a bilateral central PE, with signs of right ventricular dysfunction.

Note: Top left: Signs of right ventricular dysfunction, with dilatation of the right ventricle and septal flattening. Top right: Central PE in the right pulmonary artery. Bottom left: PE in the right pulmonary artery, extending in the segmental branches of the right lung. Bottom right: Central PE in the left pulmonary artery, extending in the segmental branches of the left lung.

Ventilation–perfusion lung scan

Ventilation–perfusion (VQ) lung scanning was the imaging method of choice to replace PA for many years, until CTPA scanning became widely available. This technique is based on the principle of "mismatch" between perfusion and ventilation, and combines perfusion scans with ventilation studies, for which multiple radiolabelled tracers are used. Typically, in patients with PE, the affected area is hypoperfused while ventilation is unaltered (VQ mismatch). Test results of lung scintigraphy can be classified in three categories: normal, high-probability, and non-diagnostic. A truly normal VQ scan safely excludes the diagnosis of PE and the sensitivity of lung scintigraphy is thus very high. But whereas a high-probability VQ scan is diagnostic of PE, VQ scanning is associated with a high number of non-diagnostic or inconclusive test results (in about 28–46% of the cases). The prevalence of PE in patients with inconclusive test results ranges from 10% to 40% and thus additional testing is needed. This drawback resulted in the reduction in the utilisation of lung scintigraphy.

Single-photon emission computed tomography

The traditional VQ scan is based on a two-dimensional image acquisition. With the use of single-photon emission CT (SPECT), the VQ scan has undergone a transition to a three-dimensional plane. The SPECT technique presumably improves the diagnostic accuracy of VQ scintigraphy, but formal outcome studies in patients with acute PE are scarce. SPECT has a lower radiation burden compared to CTPA, and available studies suggest that SPECT is associated with a lower rate of inconclusive test results (between 0% and 5%) than the traditional VQ scan, which makes it a possible promising technique. Nonetheless, large prospective outcome studies are needed to validate SPECT in patients with suspected PE.

In conclusion, CTPA and VQ scans have both been validated in strong prospective management outcome studies and are both established diagnostic imaging tests for suspected PE. At the moment, CTPA is the first choice imaging test for suspected PE, as it has several advantages over VQ: (1) it is widely available (24/7 in most centres); (2) it has an excellent diagnostic accuracy with less inconclusive test results (reported to be around 3–5%); (3) a faster acquisition time; and (4) CTPA scans may provide an alternative diagnosis if PE is ruled out. On the other hand, VQ scans are relatively inexpensive and importantly, use a lower radiation dose and do not require contrast material injection, which is preferable in patients with for instance contrast material allergies or severe renal failure. Note that CTPA is relatively contraindicated in patients with severe renal impairment. Of note, some argue to perform compression ultrasound (CUS) of the legs in the diagnostic management of suspected PE, as PE typically originates from a DVT in the lower limb and CUS does not involve radiation exposure or contrast material injection. Although in a positive CUS wave the need for further testing forms an indication for anticoagulant therapy, sensitivity of CUS for suspected PE is low (around 40%) and additional chest imaging is absolutely necessary after a negative CUS. Still, CUS could be beneficial in patients with concurrent symptoms of DVT and CT contraindications.

Challenges in Specific Patient Populations

Elderly patients

The incidence of VTE increases exponentially with age, and consequently, the majority of VTE events occur in older adults. Unfortunately, these elderly patients, with prevalent cardiopulmonary comorbidities, often present with more non-specific symptoms of PE. Moreover, elderly patients often have renal insufficiency and are thus prone to develop contrast material-induced complications after CTPA. But at the same time, the ability to exclude PE without imaging in elderly patients is diminished, because of the physiological increase in D-dimer levels with age.

Whether CDRs perform differently in elderly patients is not completely clear, but the available (mostly small retrospective) studies that compared the Wells rule with the revised Geneva score, showed superiority of the Wells rule for assessing CPTP in elderly patients, which could may be explained by the absence of the item "immobility for reasons other than surgery or fracture" in the revised Geneva score.

Given the physiological increase in D-dimer levels in older patients, the use of adapted D-dimer thresholds seems beneficial. In a large individual patient data meta-analysis (IPDMA) on diagnostic strategies for ruling out PE across different patient subgroups, it was shown that with these adapted D-dimer thresholds the proportion of elderly patients (≥80 years old) that could be excluded from having PE without imaging increased by four-fold (from ~5% to 20%). This increase in efficiency in the oldest patients was however accompanied by predicted failure rates between 2% and 4% and also with wide confidence margins.

Unfortunately, available guidelines do not provide specific recommendations on the best diagnostic approach for suspected PE in elderly patients and only include the general statement that adapted D-dimer thresholds can be used as an alternative to the fixed D-dimer threshold. Nonetheless, we suggest using these adapted D-dimer thresholds as they improve the yield of the CDR/D-dimer test combination in elderly patients considerably, which is beneficial as this limits the need for imaging tests.

Patients with cancer

Cancer patients have a four- to seven-fold increased risk for developing VTE, compared to non-cancer patients. But the clinical utility of the traditional diagnostic approach, consisting of CDRs and D-dimer testing, appears doubtful in these patients. First of all, the most commonly used CDRs include the item of active malignancy in their scores, which already increases the CPTP in these patients. Second, D-dimer levels are often increased in patients with cancer, in the absence of thrombosis, again limiting the ability of D-dimer testing to rule out PE without imaging. Consequently, the standard approach in cancer patients with suspected PE often includes performing imaging right away, without CPTP and D-dimer testing.

Whereas the adapted D-dimer thresholds have partially counteracted the reduced efficiency of D-dimer testing in cancer patients, uncertainty remains about the safety of such an approach in these patients. Previous studies showed that efficiency could be increased from about 10% — when using a fixed D-dimer threshold — up to 20–25% with adapted D-dimer thresholds, but this was associated with somewhat higher failure rates in the subgroup of cancer patients (YEARS study: failure rate 2.6% and IPDMA: failure rates between 2% and 4%). Still, we believe that these failure rates, that exceed the recent recommended margin of 2% by ISTH standards, do not indicate that these strategies are unsafe in high risk patients *per se*. First of all, as cancer patients have many persistent risk factors for PE, this will presumably lead to an increased failure rate of the strategy. But these "failures" will not necessarily be true failures of the diagnostic strategy at baseline, as some of these will likely be new thrombotic events, unrelated to the index presentation. Second, the failure rate measurement only includes patients that were managed without imaging, and as the adapted D-dimer thresholds refer fewer patients for imaging, more patients will be included in the failure rate analysis. Consequently, more failures within these adapted D-dimer strategies will be observed.

To provide a definite answer, a randomised controlled trial in patients with cancer and clinically suspected PE is currently ongoing. In this randomised study, the safety and efficiency of management by the YEARS algorithm will directly be compared against management by CTPA alone. In the meantime, current guidelines do not present clear recommendations on the best diagnostic approach for suspected PE in cancer patients, but given all these arguments, we suggest to use these adapted D-dimer thresholds as they reduce the need for imaging, which will result in less contrast material-induced complications, reduction of potentially irrelevant subsegmental emboli detection, and lower healthcare costs.

Pregnant patients

Pregnant patients have a four- to five-fold increased risk for developing VTE, compared to non-pregnant women of the same age. But despite this increased risk, the absolute risk of PE during pregnancy is modest. Nonetheless, clinicians generally use a low threshold to test for PE, due to the well-known risks of missing a PE diagnosis during pregnancy. This is illustrated by the low proportion of confirmed PE cases among pregnant patients investigated for the disease, which is about 4%.

The diagnostic approach for suspected PE during pregnancy is further complicated by the rise in D-dimer levels during pregnancy, and concerns about radiation exposure and unwanted side effects to mother and foetus when imaging is necessary. Whereas adapted D-dimer thresholds were validated in the general patient population, pregnant patients were often excluded from these studies. Hence, evidence on the use of diagnostic strategies for suspected PE in pregnant patients was lacking, until recently.

Two large prospective management studies have validated a diagnostic strategy for suspected PE in pregnancy (the CT-PE study: evaluated the revised Geneva score; and the Artemis study: evaluated the YEARS algorithm). Both studies used a pregnancy adapted diagnostic strategy, with the integration of CUS of the legs within their study protocol. With CUS, the goal was to avoid chest imaging in patients with confirmed DVT. Results showed that the yield of CUS when performing it within the diagnostic management of suspected PE was low during pregnancy, especially in patients without symptoms of DVT. But more importantly, both studies showed that pre-test probability assessment and D-dimer tests were able to safely rule out PE in pregnancy. This diagnostic approach is now supported by the latest guideline recommendation from the ESC 2019. Additionally, despite the concerns on radiation exposure in pregnant patients, more recent studies have now provided reassuring results: maternal and foetal risks are similarly low after VQ and CTPA, so both tests can safely be used when necessary.

Patients with COVID-19

COVID-19 patients are known to be at high risk for venous thrombotic events, especially but not exclusively when admitted to the ICU. The most frequent thrombotic complication in these patients is PE. Yet, clinicians face many difficulties when deciding on the best diagnostic approach for COVID-19 patients with suspected PE. First, there is a wide overlap between symptoms associated with COVID-19 and symptoms associated with PE. This challenges the question when to suspect PE in a patient with COVID-19. Second, D-dimer levels are frequently elevated in COVID-19 patients in the absence of thrombosis. Third, evidence on the use of diagnostic strategies for suspected PE in the setting of COVID-19 are scarce. And fourth, performing chest imaging may not always be feasible in the case of hemodynamic or respiratory instability.

Meanwhile, a prospective cohort study evaluating a diagnostic strategy in patients with COVID-19 has been performed. This study evaluated the YEARS algorithm in patients with suspected and confirmed COVID-19 and clinically suspected PE and results showed that CTPA could be avoided in 29% of the patients managed by YEARS, in the presence of an acceptably low failure rate. The use of diagnostic strategies in the setting of COVID-19 is also supported by current international consensus documents. We propose that strategies with adapted D-dimer thresholds are preferable, since D-dimer levels are known to be elevated in these patients and applying a fixed D-dimer threshold of 500 μg/L limits the ability to exclude PE without imaging. Still, in the previously mentioned prospective study, a high failure rate was observed in patients with a negative CTPA at baseline. This finding reflects the high thrombotic risk of these patients and new diagnostic tests should thus be initiated when symptoms progress or persist.

Conclusion

The diagnostic approach for suspected PE in haemodynamically stable patients should always start with clinical pre-test probability assessment, using validated CDRs, and D-dimer testing, even in special patient populations. This recommendation is broadly supported by the international guidelines on diagnosis of acute PE. Preferably, we recommend the use of strategies with adapted D-dimer thresholds, for obvious reasons of efficacy. Finally, as the benefit of these strategies is mostly dependent on optimal adherence, we advise to standardise a particular strategy in each individual hospital.

Bibliography

Dronkers, C.E.A. *et al.* (2017). Towards a tailored diagnostic standard for future diagnostic studies in pulmonary embolism: Communication from the SSC of the ISTH, *Journal of Thrombosis and Haemostasis*, 15(5), pp. 1040–1043.

Huisman, M.V., Barco, S., Cannegieter, S.C. *et al.* (2018). Pulmonary embolism, *Nature Reviews Disease Primers*, 4, pp. 18028.

Kearon, C. *et al.* (2019). Diagnosis of pulmonary embolism with D-dimer adjusted to clinical probability, *New England Journal of Medicine*, 381(22), pp. 2125–2134.

Konstantinides, S.V., Meyer, G., Becattini, C. *et al.* (2019). ESC guidelines for the diagnosis and management of acute pulmonary embolism developed in collaboration with the European Respiratory Society (ERS), *European Heart Journal*, 41, pp. 543–603.

Lim, W., Le Gal, G., Bates, S.M. *et al.* (2018). American society of hematology 2018 guidelines for management of venous thromboembolism: Diagnosis of venous thromboembolism, *Blood Advances*, 2(22), pp. 3226–3256.

Righini, M. *et al.* (2014). Age-adjusted D-dimer cutoff levels to rule out pulmonary embolism: The ADJUST-PE study, *JAMA*, 311(11), pp. 1117–1124.

Righini, M. *et al.* (2018). Diagnosis of pulmonary embolism during pregnancy: A multicenter prospective management outcome study, *Annals of Internal Medicine*, 169(11), pp. 766–773.

Stals, M.A.M. *et al.* (2021). Ruling out pulmonary embolism in patients with (suspected) COVID-19 — A prospective cohort study, *TH Open*, 5(3), pp. e387–e399.

Stals, M.A.M., Takada, T., Kraaijpoel, N. *et al.* (2022). Safety and efficiency of diagnostic strategies for ruling out pulmonary embolism in clinically relevant patient subgroups: A systematic review and individual-patient data meta-analysis, *Annals of Internal Medicine*, 175(2), pp. 244–255.

van der Hulle, T. *et al.* (2017). YEARS study group. Simplified diagnostic management of suspected pulmonary embolism (the YEARS study): A prospective, multicentre, cohort study, *Lancet*, 15, 390(10091): pp. 289–297.

van der Pol, L.M. *et al.* (2019). Pregnancy-adapted YEARS algorithm for diagnosis of suspected pulmonary embolism, *New England Journal of Medicine*, 380(12), pp. 1139–1149.

Van Es, E.N. *et al.* (2016). Wells rule and D-dimer testing to rule out pulmonary embolism: A systematic review and individual-patient data meta-analysis, *Annals of Internal Medicine*, 165(4), pp. 253–261.

Chapter 2

Correct Risk Stratification at Diagnosis — Why It Matters?

Mariana Pfeferman and Gregory Piazza

Division of Cardiovascular Medicine, Brigham and Women's Hospital, Harvard Medical School, Boston, MA, USA

Abstract

PE clinical presentation comprises a wide spectrum of prognoses and risk of adverse outcomes. A subset of patients, who are haemodynamically stable on presentation, may develop abrupt deterioration, despite therapeutic anticoagulation. Diagnosis of pulmonary embolism (PE) should be accompanied by risk stratification, to identify vulnerable patients who may benefit from more intensive monitoring and advanced therapies, including reperfusion. Integration of bedside scoring systems for clinical prognosis such as Pulmonary Embolism Severity Index (PESI), risk categorisation, cardiac biomarkers such as troponin, and evidence of RV dysfunction by either CT or echocardiography avoids risk misclassification and encourages evidence-based management. According to 2019 ESC Guidelines only low-risk patients with reliable medical follow-up can be treated as outpatients. Intermediate low, intermediate high-, and high-risk PE should all be hospitalised. Intermediate-high patients should be monitored closely, and the rescue reperfusion should be considered. High-risk patients should receive reperfusion treatment and haemodynamic support.

Clinical Case

A 72-year-old man with obesity, type 2 diabetes, hypertension, and hyper-lipidaemia was presented to the Emergency Department with sudden-onset chest pain, dyspnoea, and light-headedness. He recently was diagnosed with right-sided plantar fasciitis, had been wearing a walking boot, and was much more sedentary. On physical examination, he was tachycardic to 130 beats per minute, normotensive with a blood pressure of 110/72 mmHg, and hypoxemic to 90% on room air. He had clear lungs, a tachycardic rhythm, and 2+ edema of the right ankle and shin. His ECG showed sinus tachycardia at 128 beats per minute and precordial T wave inversions. His cardiac troponin was mildly increased. A chest computed tomogram was performed and demonstrated bilateral pulmonary embo-lism (PE) and evidence of right ventricular (RV) enlargement (Figure 1). The Emergency Medicine team consulted the hospital multidisciplinary PE response team with the following questions:

(1) How should the patient's risk for adverse outcomes be classified?
(2) Does the patient's risk for adverse outcomes warrant therapy beyond anticoagulation alone?

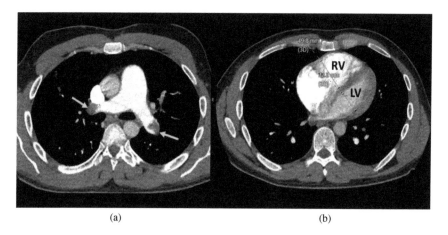

(a)   (b)

Figure 1.   72-year-old man with obesity, type 2 diabetes, hypertension, and hyperlipidemia was presented with sudden-onset chest pain, dyspnoea, and light-headedness and found to have acute bilateral pulmonary embolism (PE) (Panel a, arrows) and right ventricular (RV) enlargement (Panel b) as demonstrated by an RV-to-left ventricular (LV) diameter ratio greater than 0.9 on contrast-enhanced chest computed tomography (CT).

Clinical Clues

While symptoms and signs are critical for the prompt diagnosis of PE, they may also provide clues to the patient's risk for adverse clinical outcomes. The presence of profound dyspnoea, syncope, or cyanosis can herald a high-risk PE, whereas pleuritic pain, cough, or haemoptysis can correlate with smaller peripherally located PE. Clues to right-heart failure include tachycardia, distended jugular veins, an accentuated sound of pulmonic valve closure (P2), and a tricuspid regurgitation murmur.

Risk Scores

Because synthesising clinical indicators, laboratory testing, and imaging parameters can be challenging for even the most seasoned clinicians, risk scores have been validated to help clinicians identify patients at risk for complications who may benefit from advanced therapies beyond anticoagulation. While all risk scores aim to inform prognosis, applications can be different for each one. Some of them are used to identify patients who would be eligible for outpatient treatment, like the HESTIA decision rule. Others aim to identify patients who are at high risk for deterioration and would benefit from advanced therapies, like the Pulmonary Embolism Severity Index (PESI), simplified PESI (sPESI), and BOVA scores. The HESTIA rule comprises parameters that preclude eligibility for outpatient treatment, with the presence of some additional criteria when compared with PESI and sPESI scores, like medical or social reasons, for in-hospital treatment. The BOVA score, on the other hand, uses fewer criteria overall, but includes imaging studies and cardiac biomarker in the parameters (Table 1).

Electrocardiography

The electrocardiogram (ECG) in acute PE is typically most helpful for identification of alternative diagnoses to PE. However, the ECG can, in some cases, provide a clue to RV strain. In PE patients, the classic ECG findings of RV strain include the S1Q3T3 pattern, which shows S wave in lead I and a Q wave and T wave inversions in lead III, incomplete or complete right bundle branch block (RBBB), and T wave inversions in the anterior precordial leads.

Table 1.   Acute pulmonary embolism risk scores.

	Criteria		Advantages	Disadvantages
PESI	Age (years)	Number of years	• No need of	• Large number
	Male gender	10 pts	imaging	of variables to
	History of cancer	30 pts	studies or	consider
	Heart failure	10 pts	cardiac	• It does not
	Chronic lung disease	10 pts	biomarkers	consider signs
	Pulse ≥110/min	20 pts	• Five	of RV
	Systolic blood pressure	30 pts	classification	dysfunction
	<100 mmHg		categories	and
	Respiratory rate ≥30/min	20 pts	highlight a	myocardial
	Temperature <36°C	20 pts	broad	necrosis
	Altered mental status	60 pts	spectrum of	
	Arterial oxygen saturation	20 pts	PE-related	
	<90%		outcomes	
	Class I	**<65 pts**		
	Class II	**65–85 pts**		
	I and II: Low-risk			
	Class III	**86–105 pts**		
	III: Intermediate-risk			
	Class IV	**106–125 pts**		
	Class V	**>125 pts**		
	IV and V: High-risk			
sPESI	Age >80 years	1 pt	• Limited	• Only 2
	History of cancer	1 pt	number of	classification
	History of chronic	1 pt	variables to	categories,
	cardiopulmonary disease		consider	dichotomizing
	Heart rate ≥110 beats/	1 pt	• No need of	a wide
	minute		imaging	spectrum of
	Systolic blood pressure	1 pt	studies of	patients
	<100 mmHg		cardiac	• It does not
	Oxyhemoglobin saturation	1 pt	biomarkers	consider signs
	level <90%			of RV
				dysfunction
	Low risk	**0 pts**		and
	High risk	**≥1 pt**		myocardial
				necrosis

Table 1.   (*Continued*)

	Criteria		Advantages	Disadvantages
HESTIA rule	Hemodynamic instability	1 pt	• Considers social reasons for in-hospital treatment	• Large number of variables to consider
	Thrombolysis or embolectomy indicated	1 pt		• Considers pain, which can be a highly subjective criterion and limits assessment in patients who cannot express symptoms
	Active bleeding or high risk of bleeding	1 pt	• Well-validates for assessment of outpatient treatment of PE	
	Need for supplemental oxygen	1 pt		
	PE diagnosed during anticoagulant treatment	1 pt		
	Severe pain requiring intravenous medications	1 pt		• Only 2 classification categories, dichotomizing a wide spectrum of patients
	Medical or social reason for in-hospital treatment	1 pt		
	Severe renal or liver impairment	1 pt		
	Pregnancy	1 pt		
	Documented history of heparin-induced thrombocytopenia	1 pt		
	Eligible for outpatient treatment	**0 pts**		
	Not eligible for outpatient treatment	**≥1 pt**		
BOVA score	Systolic blood pressure 90–100 mm Hg	2 pts	• It considers signs of RV dysfunction and myocardial necrosis	• Need of imaging study and cardiac biomarker
	Cardiac troponin elevation	2 pts		
	Right ventricular dysfunction (echocardiogram or CT scan)	2 pts	• Limited number of variables to consider	
	Heart rate ≥110 beats per minute	1 pt		
	Risk stage I	**0–2 pts**		
	Risk stage II	**3–4 pts**		
	Risk stage III	**>4 pts**		

Laboratory Studies

Cardiac biomarkers

The cardiac biomarkers, such as troponin, brain-type natriuretic peptide (BNP), N-terminal (NT)-pro hormone BNP (NT-pro-BNP), and heart-type fatty acid-binding protein (H-FABP) are indicators of RV dysfunction and can aid in risk stratification of PE patients. The elevations in cardiac troponin and BNP or NT-pro-BNP result from RV microinfarction and increased RV shear stress, respectively, reflecting the sequela of RV pressure overload. On their own, elevations in troponin and BNP or NT-pro-BNP have limited specificity and positive predictive value for early mortality in normotensive patients. However, when analysed in combination with clinical and imaging findings, troponin, in particular, may improve the identification of an elevated risk PE, while BNP or NT-pro-BNP have a high sensitivity and negative predictive value, excluding unfavourable early clinical outcomes when negative. Increased troponin and BNP are associated with higher short-term mortality and adverse outcomes in patients with acute PE. Additionally, among normotensive patients, cardiac biomarkers distinguish intermediate-risk from low-risk PE.

Imaging Studies

Chest computed tomography

Chest computed tomography (CT) is the standard diagnostic imaging exam to detect or exclude PE. However, contrast-enhanced chest CT is also an important instrument in the detection of RV enlargement. It is an especially convenient risk stratification tool because it utilises the same data from an initial diagnostic study. Based on measurements from the axial CT view, RV enlargement, defined as a ratio of RV to left ventricle (LV) greater than 0.9 (Figure 2), has been found to be a significant independent predictor of PE-related mortality at 30 days.

Echocardiography

While the echocardiogram lacks sensitivity as a diagnostic tool for PE, it is a key component in risk stratification due to its accuracy in detecting RV dysfunction. It should be considered in patients with acute PE and clinical evidence of RV failure, elevated cardiac biomarkers, suspected arterial

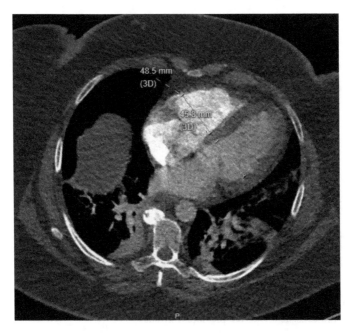

Figure 2. Contrast-enhanced chest computed tomogram (CT) demonstrating right ventricular (RV) enlargement as defined by an increased RV diameter-to-left ventricular (LV) diameter ratio (4.85 cm/4.58 cm = 1.0; normal ≤ 0.9).

hypotension, clinical deterioration, or suspicion of other comorbid cardiac disease. RV dysfunction is evidenced in the echocardiogram by RV dilation and hypokinesis (a consequence of the increased pulmonary vascular resistance), interventricular septal deviation towards the left ventricle (LV), and abnormal LV filling (Figure 3). Impaired LV filling on echocardiography and consequent decreased left-sided cardiac output can result in systemic arterial hypotension, coronary artery hypoperfusion, and RV ischemia. Recently, a systematic approach to echocardiographic assessment, including evaluation of several parameters of RV structure and function, has been recommended over a limited evaluation of RV size and contractility.

An Integrated Approach to Risk Stratification

PE clinical presentation comprises a wide spectrum of prognosis and risk of adverse outcomes. A subset of patients, who are haemodynamically

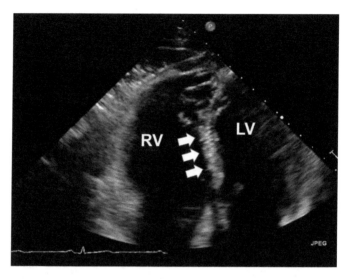

Figure 3. Transthoracic echocardiogram, apical four-chamber view, demonstrating right ventricular (RV) dilation, with interventricular septum deviation toward the left ventricle (LV) (arrows), consistent with RV pressure overload.

stable on presentation, may develop abrupt deterioration, despite therapeutic anticoagulation. These patients may progress to severe hypoxemia, cardiogenic shock, systemic arterial hypotension, and sudden death. As soon as PE is suspected, the diagnosis confirmation should be accompanied by risk stratification, to identify vulnerable patients who would benefit from more intensive monitoring and potentially, advanced therapies. A diagnostic algorithm (Figure 4) integrating clinical prognostic indicators, cardiac biomarkers, and evidence of RV dysfunction detected by either CT scan or echocardiography provides the best pathway for more precise and individualised management of the risk of adverse outcomes.

A number of risk stratification strategies have been proposed in the literature. The 2019 European Society of Cardiology (ESC) Guidelines classifies patients into four categories of risk for early mortality: low, intermediate-low, intermediate-high, and high-risk PE. High-risk PE is marked by haemodynamic instability. Intermediate-high risk PE patients are characterised by a high PESI or sPESI score, RV dysfunction on imaging and signs of myocardial necrosis, with the difference that high risk patients are haemodynamically unstable, with shock or hypotension.

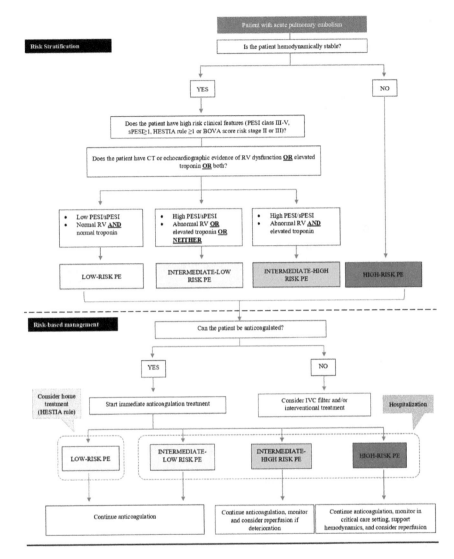

Figure 4. Approach to risk stratification and risk-based management of acute pulmonary embolism.

Notes: CT: computed tomography; IVC: inferior vena cava; PE: Pulmonary Embolism Severity Index; sPESI: simplified Pulmoanry Embolism Severity Index; RV: right ventricular.

Intermediate-low risk patients are haemodynamically stable and also have high PESI or sPESI score but may have either RV dysfunction or myocardial necrosis or neither. Lastly, low risk patients are haemodynamically stable, have low PESI or sPESI and have no signs of RV dysfunction and myocardial necrosis.

In contrast, the American Heart Association has classified PE into three categories: low risk, submassive and massive. However, the criteria used for the classification are similar: haemodynamic status, PESI or sPESI and evidence of RV dysfunction by either imaging or troponin. Massive PE is characterised by unstable haemodynamic status. Submassive PE patients also have high PESI or sPESI scores, are haemodynamically stable, and have evidence of RV dysfunction by imaging or biomarker. On the other hand, low risk patients are haemodynamically stable, with PESI or sPESI and no evidence of RV dysfunction. The submassive category from the AHA may be challenging as it comprises a heterogeneous population, with different risk levels. Considering that, the ESC stratified this category into intermediate-low and intermediate-high risks, which is the main difference between the two risk classifications.

Multidisciplinary PE Response Team Role in Risk Stratification

The risk stratification criteria to identify patients who would benefit from advanced therapies can vary among clinicians but does not demonstrate as much variability as treatment strategies. The lack of comparative studies to guide the large number of treatments available for PE and limited guideline recommendations, prompted a movement towards gathering different perspectives and expertise from different medical and surgical specialties in the approach to PE patients. To provide more individualised risk stratification and therapy in the absence of definitive randomised trial data and clear evidence-based guideline recommendations, multidisciplinary PE response teams emerged to meet the need for expert PE care. This team approach helps to balance the benefits of intervention against potential risks of cardiopulmonary failure, haemodynamic instability, or death, also avoiding biases from individual specialties or individual practitioners in planning therapeutic strategy.

The Impact of Risk Stratification on Decision-Making

Identified patients who would benefit from advanced therapies, the final step is to establish the best management and choose the best treatment aiming to avoid abrupt deteriorations. According to the 2019 ESC

Guidelines for diagnosis and management of acute PE, only low-risk PE patients with reliable medical follow-up can be discharged home on anti-coagulation without hospitalisation. Patients with intermediate low-, intermediate high-, and high-risk PE should all be hospitalised. Intermediate-high patients should be monitored closely, and the rescue reperfusion should be considered if they deteriorate despite anticoagulation. High-risk PE patients should be considered for early reperfusion treatment with or without by haemodynamic support.

Clinical Case

(1) This patient has an increased sPESI or PESI score with signs of RV dysfunction by CT and myocardial necrosis and ischemia by troponin and ECG (T wave inversions). Considering that, his PE would be classified as intermediate-high risk.
(2) The patient should continue anticoagulation and close monitoring and, in case of deterioration, should be considered for reperfusion.

Conclusion

- Risk stratification is a fundamental step seeking to identify vulnerable patients, who may abruptly deteriorate despite anticoagulation.
- Integration of clinical prognostic indicators, risk categorisation, cardiac biomarkers, and evidence of RV dysfunction by either CT or echocardiography avoid risk underestimation and leads to the correct management.
- According to 2019 ESC guidelines only low risk patients with reliable medical follow-up can be treated as outpatients. Intermediate low, intermediate high- and high-risk PE should all be hospitalised. Intermediate-high patients should be monitored closely, and the rescue reperfusion should be considered. High-risk patients should receive reperfusion treatment and haemodynamic support.

Bibliography

Barnes, G.D., Muzikansky, A., Cameron, S., Giri, J., Heresi, G.A., Jaber, W. *et al.* Comparison of 4 acute pulmonary embolism mortality risk scores in patients evaluated by pulmonary embolism response teams, *JAMA Network Open*, 3(8), pp. 2010779.

Goldhaber, S.Z. (2002). Echocardiography in the management of pulmonary embolism, *Annals of Internal Medicine*, 136, pp. 691–700.

Goldhaber, S.Z. and Elliott, C.G. (2003). Acute pulmonary embolism: Part II: Risk stratification, treatment, and prevention, *Circulation*, 108, pp. 2834–2838.

Hendriks, S.V., den Exter, P.L., Zondag, W., Brouwer, R., Eijsvogel, M., Grootenboers, M.J. *et al*. Reasons for hospitalization of patients with acute pulmonary embolism based on the hestia decision rule, *Thrombosis and Haemostasis,* 120(8), pp. 1217–1220.

Jaff, M.R., McMurtry, M.S., Archer, S.L., Cushman, M., Goldenberg, N., Goldhaber, S.Z. *et al*. Management of massive and submassive pulmonary embolism, iliofemoral deep vein thrombosis, and chronic thromboembolic pulmonary hypertension: A scientific statement from the American Heart Association, *Circulation*, 123(16), pp. 1788–1830.

Jiménez, D., Aujesky, D., Moores, L., Gómez, V., Lobo, J.L., Uresandi, F. *et al*. (2010). Simplification of the pulmonary embolism severity index for prognostication in patients with acute symptomatic pulmonary embolism, *Archives of Internal Medicine*, 170(15), pp. 1383–1389.

Kucher, N. and Goldhaber, S.Z. (2003). Cardiac biomarkers for risk stratification of patients with acute pulmonary embolism, *Circulation*, 2003, 108(18), pp. 2191–2194.

Piazza, G. (2020). Advanced management of intermediate- and high-risk pulmonary embolism: JACC Focus Seminar, *Journal of the American College of Cardiology*, 76, pp. 2117–2127.

Piazza, G. and Goldhaber, S.Z. (2006). Acute pulmonary embolism — Part I: Epidemiology and diagnosis, Vol. 114, *Circulation*. Lippincott Williams & Wilkins.

Provias, T., Dudzinski, D.M., Jaff, M.R., Rosenfield, K., Channick, R., Baker, J. *et al*. (1995). The Massachusetts General Hospital Pulmonary Embolism Response Team (MGH PERT): Creation of a multidisciplinary program to improve care of patients with massive and submassive pulmonary embolism, *Hospital Practice*, 42(1), pp. 31–37.

Todoran, T.M., Giri, J., Barnes, G.D., Rosovsky, R.P., Chang, Y., Jaff, M.R. *et al*. (2018). Treatment of submassive and massive pulmonary embolism: A clinical practice survey from the second annual meeting of the Pulmonary Embolism Response Team Consortium, *Journal of Thrombosis and Thrombolysis*, 46(1), pp. 39–49.

Zondag, W., Mos, I.C.M., Creemers-Schild, D., Hoogerbrugge, A.D.M., Dekkers, O.M., Dolsma, J. *et al*. (2011). Outpatient treatment in patients with acute pulmonary embolism: The Hestia Study, *Journal of Thrombosis and Haemostasis*, 9(8), pp. 1500–1507.

Chapter 3

Outpatient Management of Pulmonary Embolism: Who Can I Send Home?

Bavithra Vijayakumar* and Chris Davies†

**Royal Brompton and Harefield Hospitals, Guy's and
St Thomas' NHS Foundation Trust, London, UK*

*†Department of Respiratory Medicine, University Hospitals
Dorset NHS Trust, UK*

Abstract

Pulmonary embolism is a major cause of morbidity and mortality across the globe, but there is growing evidence that outpatient management can be a safe option for some patients, thus reducing risks associated with a prolonged hospital stay. However, careful risk stratification is essential in order to appropriately select patients suitable for outpatient management. This chapter summarises the various risk-stratification methods clinicians can use to aid decision-making, including clinical presentation, validated risk-prediction tools, methods of assessing co-existent right heart dysfunction, as well as summarising two national guidelines: British Thoracic Society and European Society of Cardiology guidelines. In addition, this chapter gives practical advice on management in difficult scenarios, such as pulmonary embolism in pregnancy, and concludes with worked clinical examples to consolidate the theory taught and allow readers to practise application of these tools to clinical scenarios.

Introduction: Defining Outpatient

When considering patients suitable for outpatient management, there is a requirement to define outpatient. This will depend on different healthcare settings and in our view usually refers to patients leaving hospital to return to their home or place of residence, but it is recognised that there are other models for early discharge, which may include use of early discharge facilities or medical hotels. These can still allow patients access to healthcare support outside of an acute hospital setting. This chapter refers to the identification of patients with PE who can leave hospital with treatment and return to their home environment, and who have been assessed as safe to do so by experienced clinicians.

Why Manage Patients with PE as an Outpatient?

Venous thromboembolism (VTE) is one of the most frequent causes of cardiovascular mortality, which includes myocardial infarction and stroke, but with growing evidence of the safety outcomes of early discharge and the development of direct oral anticoagulants (DOACs), outpatient management of selected patients has become a safe and feasible option. This approach began at first in the 1990s after successful introduction of safe outpatient pathways for patients with confirmed and/or suspected deep vein thrombosis (DVT) using low molecular weight heparin (LMWH), avoiding admission for the majority, with consequent cost and bed savings. It soon became apparent that there may be a cohort of "low risk" patients with PE where clinicians did not see or anticipate a complicated course during hospital admission.

The average length of stay for a pulmonary embolism (PE) admission varies depending on clinical factors but in many observational studies for relatively straightforward cases was still approximately 13 days in 2001, dropping to 9 days in 2013, and during which time patients were effectively anticoagulated and observed, most requiring no other significant interventions. The RIETE registry has shown significant temporal changes in the management of PE over time, coinciding with a time when there has been an increase in the use of LMWH and DOACs, with an increasing guideline-based approach, also associated with a reduction in mortality.

The benefits of outpatient management are obvious and parallel to other pathways for ambulatory acute care and include reduced length of hospital stay with associated reduction in costs, reduction in morbidity and mortality associated with hospital-acquired infections, and improvement in health-related quality of life. Although experienced clinicians may consider they can subjectively identify patients who may be safely managed at home with PE, the additional use of risk-stratification scores and guidance allows careful selection of patients suitable for safe early outpatient management, and also aids recognition of those who would be best managed, at least initially, as an inpatient.

Risk Stratification

Although the majority of patients presenting with acute PE have no or few complications, a proportion have PE-associated morbidity (such as bleeding associated with anticoagulation) and some may die. Therefore, careful risk-stratification is required to ensure patient safety.

Clinical presentation

The commonest clinical presentations of a PE are that of chest pain, breathlessness, and cough, with symptoms usually presenting when more than 50% of the pulmonary vasculature is occluded depending on comorbidities and cardiorespiratory reserve. Severe pleuritic pain, haemoptysis, and occasionally fever may be encountered in the presence of a pulmonary infarct, which is usually due to the presence of peripheral thrombus. To aid decision-making about early discharge, a careful history should be taken to elicit and rule out symptoms of pre-syncope or syncope, which are associated with higher 30-day mortality and which would warrant initial inpatient treatment and monitoring. Additionally, patients may complain of retrosternal, angina-like pain due to right ventricular ischaemia if a large and/or central PE is present and again, we would recommend initial inpatient management, even if risk stratification using scoring systems suggests a low-risk PE.

Risk scores

There are a variety of validated scores that exists (Chapter 2, Table 1), which can be used for these purposes in PE patients.

Pulmonary Embolism Severity Index (PESI) and simplified PESI (sPESI)

The Pulmonary Embolism Severity Index (PESI) and simplified PESI (sPESI) scores use a combination of demographic data, patient comorbidities, and clinical parameters to calculate a 30-day mortality risk, with a patient in PESI class 1 (very low risk) or class II (low risk) having a 30-day mortality risk of <1.6% and 3.6%, respectively, and with a low risk of recurrent VTE or major bleeding events during the follow up period of 30 days.

The sPESI is a derivative of the PESI score and is easier to calculate than the PESI score. This too has been extensively validated and shown to be non-inferior to the PESI score in predicting 30-day mortality. A 30-day mortality in the low-risk group, i.e., score of 0, is around 1%. Both scores refer to "cancer" as a heavily weighted factor (30 points in PESI and 1 in sPESI) and it is considered that this refers to active cancer and/or treatment for cancer within the last 6 months and not some distant episode in a patient's medical history.

Geneva score

The Geneva score (once PE is confirmed as opposed to the pre-test proba-bility Geneva score) not only incorporates patient comorbidities with clini-cal variables but also includes assessment for leg DVT by ultrasound scanning and can help predict 90-day mortality. However, the need to include leg USS as part of the assessment may limit its usefulness in set-tings where leg USS for DVT is not a routine part of PE assessment (like the UK). Furthermore, comparison between the PESI and Geneva scores in attempting to identify the correct population for safe discharge suggests that the Geneva score might not be as effective as the PESI score, and that PESI may also identify a larger cohort suitable for outpatient management.

Hestia criteria

The Hestia criteria are a list of exclusion criteria for patients with confirmed PE, which include clinical, demographic, and comorbidity-based parameters. Validation studies suggest that patients without any of these criteria can be safely managed at home. One attraction of the Hestia score is that no addi-tional risk stratification is required as studies have shown that these criteria are robust even when considering additional markers of right ventricular (RV) strain such as echocardiography and cardiac biomarkers (see the following).

Other scores

There are a few other scores that have been assessed and proposed for PE management, including risk scores like BOVA. This four-point score uses pulse rate, blood pressure, presence of cardiac biomarkers, and RV dilatation, categorising patients into three groups, but the lowest risk group had a 4.4% risk of PE-related complications which is not as favourable as using PESI/sPESI scores or the Hestia criteria.

Raised cardiac biomarkers

There are two cardiac biomarkers available for "routine" clinical care that can be useful in the risk stratification of patients with confirmed PE. These are troponin and brain natriuretic peptides (BNP and NT-pro BNP). The underlying aetiology of a raised troponin in the context of a PE is myocardial ischaemia/necrosis, whereas BNP is likely linked to dilatation or stretch of cardiac myocytes, likely reflecting right ventricular (RV) dilatation.

The raised pressures in the pulmonary arteries (PA) due to acute clot burden, results in RV dilatation (in the absence of time to promote hypertrophy), which in turn results in reduced left ventricular filling, reduced cardiac output, and consequently myocardial ischaemia. This in turn causes further impairment of RV function and the spiral of haemodynamic collapse begins. Both raised troponin and BNP/NT pro-BNP are associated with increased mortality, and also with a more complicated clinical course and outcome (Figure 1).

Right ventricular dilatation

As described, right ventricular *dysfunction* as a consequence of severe PE is associated with the spiral of haemodynamic collapse, if untreated and

Early mortality risk		Indicators of risk			
		Haemo-dynamic instability	Clinical parameters of PE severity/comorbidity: PESI III–V or sPESI≥1	RV dysfunction on TTE or CTPA	Elevated cardiac troponin levels
High		+	(+)	+	(+)
Interme-diate	Intermediate–high	-	+	+	+
	Intermediate–low	-	+	One (or none) positive	
Low		-	-	-	Assessment optional; if assessed, negative

Figure 1. ESC guidelines on diagnosis and management of acute pulmonary embolism, 2014, *European Heart Journal.*

not adequately recognised as a risk factor, even in normotensive patients. In contrast, a normally functioning RV has a negative predictive value of 93% for all-cause mortality at 30 days.

The RV can be assessed by using CT scan images taken at the time of the CT Pulmonary Angiogram (CTPA) and/or by echocardiography. When measuring RV dysfunction using the CTPA, interobserver variability is a recognised concern and so ideally, the presence or absence of RV dilatation should be reported by Thoracic Radiologists reporting the original scan confirming the presence of PE. Hospitals should be encouraged to implement this relatively simple risk stratification into routine radiology reporting. If, however, this is not always the case, non-radiologists can with minimal training and simple instruction calculate this ratio as effectively and accurately as a Thoracic Radiologist. There is no difference between assessing RV dilatation on axial imaging versus 4-chamber imaging, and it is often evident on simple inspection of the CT scan anyway, that the RV is dilated compared to the LV indicating RV dilatation.

The suggestion is to:

(a) Measure perpendicular to the long axis at the maximum measurable diameter.
(b) Measure through to the endocardial borders of ventricles (see the following).
(c) Then calculate using the numerical values, the RV:LV ratio. The RV is considered dilated if the RV:LV ratio is >0.9.

In Figure 2, it is easy to see that the RV is dilated compared to the LV, without measuring.

RV dilatation can also be assessed by echocardiography, if available, although often this investigation requires expertise of a physiologist to perform and may need interpretation by a cardiologist, so the timing of echocardiography will depend on individual healthcare settings and may not be immediately helpful when early decisions for discharge planning are necessary in suitable patients. For this reason, when required, the CTPA is probably the best source for identifying whether there is RV dilatation.

Clinical Application of PE Guidelines

Two well-recognised guidelines that are useful for the management of PE are by the European Society of Cardiology (ESC) and British Thoracic Society (BTS).

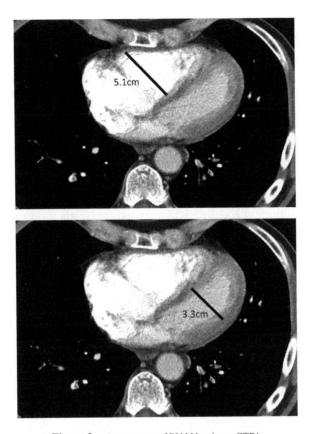

Figure 2.   Assessment of RV:LV ratio on CTPA.

In short, the British Thoracic Society recommends the use of PESI/sPESI or Hestia, and that those who have either a PESI of 1/2 or sPESI of 0 or Hestia of 0, should be considered for outpatient management. When using the BTS strategy with sPESI/PESI, a number of safety exclusion criteria is still required, including the absence of:

- Oxygen saturation <90%
- Systolic blood pressure <100 mm Hg
- Chest pain needing opiates
- Active bleeding
- High risk of bleeding (stroke within the preceding 10 days)
- Gastrointestinal bleed within the last 14 days or platelet count <75,000/mm^3

- Obesity (weight >150 kg)
- Heparin-induced thrombocytopenia
- Severe renal failure (creatinine clearance <30 mL/min)
- Therapeutic anticoagulation (international normalised ratio ≥2.0) at diagnosis
- Barriers to treatment adherence or follow-up

Because of the similarities between the exclusion criteria and Hestia, it might be considered easier to simply use the Hestia criteria in decisions about outpatient management with confirmed PE, but in the authors' experience, many clinicians seem to prefer the more objective parameters within sPESI/PESI to just using Hestia criteria alone. An additional issue is that when assessing for suitability for outpatient management, RV dilatation may not necessarily be associated with mortality if appropriate patient selection is performed using the Hestia criteria. One study showed that RV/LV ratio was not associated with all-cause mortality or adverse effects and would have excluded 30% of their cohort using Hestia criteria.

In contrast, the ESC guidelines suggest using the sPESI in conjunction with cardiac biomarker evaluation. Furthermore, clinical application of guidelines is often impacted on by clinical acumen and clinical experience and the aforementioned scores should be used to *guide* and not *replace* the clinical decision-making process. Any decision to discharge a patient home with outpatient treatment should be made by an experienced clinician. This does not necessarily need to be a doctor and may be an advanced nurse practitioner or equivalent, with training and adequate experience in managing patients with PE.

Pulmonary Infarcts and Early Discharge

Another confusing symptom is pleuritic chest pain, often with haemoptysis, with CT findings being typically a subpleural wedge-shaped infarct. Pulmonary infarcts are often seen in more peripherally sited PEs. To firmly diagnose an infarct, follow-up imaging is required as true infarct and necrosis heals with scarring, although in about 50% of patients, radiological abnormalities may resolve on follow-up imaging. A lower in-hospital and 15-day mortality rate has been noted in patients with probable infarction, especially in those with haemoptysis, and where a diagnosis of pulmonary infarct has been made based on radiological grounds, there was no difference in inpatient, 30 or 90-day mortality. Therefore, although pain can be quite severe at presentation, there is no convincing evidence that this alone is an indication to remain an inpatient, unless requiring significant analgesia or if other exclusion criteria/Hestia criteria are not met.

Approach to the Use of Cardiac Biomarkers and Measures of Right Ventricular Dilatation

If using the British Thoracic Society Guidelines with either Hestia criteria or PESI/sPESI, identification of RV dilatation (either on CTPA or echocardiogram) should then prompt the measurement of a cardiac bio-marker. If there is a positive troponin and/or BNP, then a patient who fulfils either the sPESI/PESI or Hestia criteria, but with both RV dilatation and a positive biomarker, would be advised to remain in hospital, as the combination of both risk stratification factors increases the likelihood of an unfavourable outcome. A patient with a negative biomarker should undergo clinical assessment but could still be managed as an outpatient. If a safer approach is wanted, then as per the ESC guidelines, either a posi-tive biomarker or evidence of RV dilation should prompt admission.

Unfortunately, cardiac biomarkers, like troponin are often requested and performed before the diagnosis is clear, and frequently prior to con-firmation of PE presence by imaging. The causes of a raised troponin are numerous, including sepsis and renal dysfunction, as well as myocardial injury. Therefore, the troponin result should only be interpreted in the context of a confirmed PE and will be dependent on clinician confidence and experience. Thus, sending a troponin unnecessarily can complicate decision-making about discharge.

Clot Burden and Distribution and Early Discharge

The burden of clot on CTPA at presentation can sometimes deter clini-cians from outpatient management. Although a larger clot burden has been associated with evidence of RV dilatation, it has not been shown to impact short-term mortality. Furthermore, if the clot burden is clinically significant, this is likely to be reflected in the PESI or sPESI score, thus making the patient unsuitable for early discharge.

The presence of a saddle embolus might also raise concerns about early discharge. While the presence of a saddle embolus does not infer higher inpatient mortality when compared to non-saddle embolism, the former is associated with a higher rate of respiratory failure and cardiac arrest, therefore, even with a low PESI or sPESI score, we would recommend hospital admission and a period of clinical monitoring.

Outpatient Management of PE in Pregnancy

VTE is one of the main causes of maternal death in the UK, where the Royal Society of Obstetricians & Gynaecologists guidelines provide advice on how to manage PE in pregnant individuals, but not on selection of patients suitable for outpatient management. Pregnancy is one of the exclusion criteria in the Hestia tool, therefore these patients should be managed as an inpatient, initially, and decision regarding discharge should be made by a senior decision-maker, with close input from obstetric experts to ensure the best management for both patient and baby, especially as they will require anticoagulation management approaching delivery. A similar approach may be necessary in patients who are post-partum (within a few weeks of delivery) where anticoagulation may also be challenging and when mothers will rarely want to remain in hospital when they have a newborn at home.

Clinical Cases

Case 1

A 70-year-old woman presents to the Emergency Department with a 3-day history of worsening breathlessness, with no accompanying chest pain. She is usually fit and well with no comorbidities and is on no regular medications. She lives alone and is independent of her activities of daily living. Her daughter lives nearby and is able to monitor her mother's condition if discharged home.

Clinical examination: Chest clear to auscultation. Heart rate regular 88/min, peripheral oxygen saturations 96% on room air. Blood pressure 120/60 mmHg. Clinically appears well. Blood tests taken on admission included a positive D-dimer and raised troponin at 35 (normal <14). A CTPA shows bilateral pulmonary emboli but without definite RV dilatation.

Using risk-prediction tools: Her PESI score = 2 (Class 2, low risk), sPESI score = 0 (low risk), and Hestia criteria are negative. Therefore, according to the BTS guidelines, she can be sent home. However, she has a positive/ elevated troponin suggesting a degree of RV strain, so if following the ESC guidelines, a raised troponin puts this patient at intermediate risk of mortality (i.e., 3–25% 30-day mortality) and therefore she may need to be considered for inpatient management.

Clinical course: She was kept as an inpatient overnight with cardiac monitoring, in case of PE-associated arrhythmias and the potential need for escalation of treatment, but her clinical status remained stable, and she was subsequently discharged home within 48 hours.

Caveats: A troponin level had been sent as a workup for breathlessness, as is often the case, but should only be requested after the diagnosis of PE is confirmed. In this case, the elevated troponin required the patient to remain in hospital, perhaps unnecessarily but with a good outcome.

Case 2

An 80-year-old man with lung cancer (not for further active management) attends the Emergency Department with left-sided chest pain, and is diagnosed with an acute left-sided peripheral PE. He is an ex-smoker, having stopped approximately 15 years ago, with a 30-pack year history. He is on inhalers regularly for COPD. He lives with his wife who is in good health.

He has peripheral oxygen saturations 95% on room air. Heart rate regular 80/min. Blood pressure 140/90 mmHg and temperature 37°C.

Using risk prediction tools: His sPESI score is 2 (one point for malignancy, and one point for chronic cardiopulmonary disease), and is therefore not suitable for hospital discharge. However, this score will not change with time, as his comorbidities are fixed. Determining suitability for discharge and how long to monitor as an inpatient is therefore challenging, especially since his clinical and haemodynamic status are satisfactory. However, it is well known that patients with COPD and malignancy are at higher risk of PE-associated mortality, therefore close monitoring is required until it is clear he is stable or improving. Furthermore, deterioration related to the PE may be falsely attributed to breathlessness or pain associated with the underlying comorbidities.

The authors propose the following in a case like this, as options to facilitate early discharge.

(a) Repeat PESI or sPESI at 48 hours into admission. The non-fixed variables may reduce indicating clinical improvement(s), but also may worsen indicating that early discharge is not appropriate. Thus, if clinical parameters are stable or better, early discharge can be considered, despite a high risk PESI/ sPESI.

(b) Early outpatient follow up. Clinical follow up post PE is usually recommended at 3 months post hospital discharge. But in patients in whom early discharge was facilitated but who were at higher risk, very early follow up, either over the phone or face-to-face in ambulatory care within days of discharge and repeatedly during an initial period of 1–2 weeks may further help facilitate early, but safe discharge.

Dilemmas: It is not uncommon to be faced with a clinical scenario where the patient is adamant they wish to go home, despite medical advice. For instance, in the above case where the patient is clinically well and does not comprehend the clinician's desire for them to remain an inpatient. In these situations, we would advise that the risks and benefits of inpatient versus outpatient management are carefully outlined to the patient and documented clearly in the medical casenotes. In some centres, the patient might be required to sign a "discharge against medical advice" form, but this should be left to the discretion of the senior decision-maker involved in the management and discharge of the patient.

Summary

Here we provide an insight into the application of risk-prediction tools and national guidelines that clinicians can use to appropriately select and effectively manage patients with PE in the outpatient setting. As aforementioned, these guidelines should not replace clinical reasoning and experience, but provide objective, evidence-based tools to avoid overreliance on subjective methods.

Key points:

- Patients with low PESI scores (1 and 2) or sPESI of 0 or negative Hestia criteria can be safely managed as an outpatient.

- Centres should aim for RV dilatation being reported by Radiologists, failing which, adequate training should be provided to junior doctors to calculate this independently, although there is a lack of consensus in the guidelines with regard to the clinical relevance of a dilated RV when determining suitability for outpatient management.
- Evaluation of cardiac biomarkers should be considered in patients with features of RV dilatation on CTPA or echocardiography, with inpatient management if a raised cardiac biomarker is found in addition.
- In patients with a raised PESI (3 or above) or sPESI >0 due to co-existing comorbidities, other methods of risk-stratification and early follow up should be considered, in order to facilitate earlier discharge.

Bibliography

Aujesky, D., Obrosky, D.S., Stone, R.A. *et al.* (2005). Derivation and validation of a prognostic model for pulmonary embolism, *American Journal of Respiratory and Critical Care Medicine*, 172, pp. 1041–1046.

Bova, C., Vanni, S., Prandoni, P. *et al.* (2018). A prospective validation of the Bova score in normotensive patients with acute pulmonary embolism, *Thrombosis Research*, 165, pp. 107–111.

Ende-Verhaar, Y.M., Kroft, L.J.M., Mos, I.C.M. *et al.* Accuracy and reproducibility of CT right-to-left ventricular diameter measurement in patients with acute pulmonary embolism, *PLOS ONE*, 12, pp. e0188862.

Hendriks, S.V., Klok, F.A., den Exter, P.L. *et al.* (2020). Right ventricle-to-left ventricle diameter ratio measurement seems to have no role in low-risk patients with pulmonary embolism treated at home triaged by Hestia criteria, *American Journal of Respiratory and Critical Care Medicine*, 202, pp. 138–141.

Jiménez, D. (2010). Simplification of the pulmonary embolism severity index for prognostication in patients with acute symptomatic pulmonary embolism, *Archives of Internal Medicine*, 170, pp. 1383–1389.

Jiménez, D., de Miguel-Díez, J., Guijarro, R. *et al.* (2016). Trends in the management and outcomes of acute pulmonary embolism, *Journal of the American College of Cardiology*, 67, pp. 162–170.

Jimenez, D., Diaz, G., Molina, J. *et al.* Troponin I and risk stratification of patients with acute nonmassive pulmonary embolism, *European Respiratory Journal*, 31, pp. 847–853.

Jiménez, D., Yusen, R.D., Otero, R. *et al.* (2007). Prognostic models for selecting patients with acute pulmonary embolism for initial outpatient therapy, *Chest*, 132, pp. 24–30.

Kwak, M.K., Kim, W.Y., Lee, C.W. *et al.* (2013). The impact of saddle embolism on the major adverse event rate of patients with non-high-risk pulmonary embolism, *The British Journal of Radiology*, 86, pp. 20130273.

Okushi, Y., Kusunose, K., Okayama, Y. *et al.* Acute hospital mortality of venous thromboembolism in patients with cancer from registry data, *Journal of the American Heart Association*, 10, pp. e019373.

Pathak, R., Giri, S., Aryal, M.R. *et al.* Comparison between saddle versus non-saddle pulmonary embolism: Insights from nationwide inpatient sample, *Blood*, 124, pp. 58–59.

Zondag, W., Mos, I.C.M., Creemers-Schild, D. *et al.* (2011). Outpatient treatment in patients with acute pulmonary embolism: The Hestia Study, *Journal of Thrombosis and Haemostasis*, 9, pp. 1500–1507.

Part 2

Emergencies

Chapter 4

Navigating the Acute Treatment Landscape: An Overview

Eileen Harder

Division of Pulmonary Critical Care Medicine, Brigham and Women's Hospital, Harvard Medical School, Boston, MA, USA

Abstract

Acute pulmonary embolism (PE) is a highly complex disease associated with considerable morbidity and mortality. Following diagnosis, rapid risk stratification is crucial in guiding treatment selection. While there may be a wide variety of initial presentations, the severity of disease — and therefore the risk of death — depends upon the degree of imposed right ventricular dysfunction and consequent haemodynamic impact. As such, current risk stratification algorithms focus on assessing the status of the right ventricle to group patients by disease risk and to guide early management. Immediate reperfusion is critical in the subset with haemodynamic instability, although selection of the most appropriate modality is a nuanced decision that requires special consideration in certain patients. Furthermore, while anticoagulation remains the mainstay of treatment in haemodynamically stable PE, there has been significant interest in the application of reperfusion therapies to this population. This chapter will focus on the treatment of acute PE, opening with initial risk stratification followed by the separate management of haemodynamically unstable and stable disease.

Introduction

Estimated to be the third most common cause of cardiovascular death, an acute pulmonary embolism (PE) carries significant morbidity and mortality. Given the wide array of presentations — often with non-specific symptoms — delays to diagnosis and treatment are common and are associated with worse outcomes including mortality. Beyond diagnostic algorithms, multiple systems have therefore been designed to rapidly assess mortality risk and guide early treatment decisions. This chapter will discuss the approach to management of an acute PE, with a particular focus on initial risk stratification and treatment selection.

Initial Risk Stratification

From the initial presenting symptoms to the anatomical clot features to the consequent haemodynamic insult, acute PE is a highly diverse disease. One unifying feature, however, is the pathophysiologic interaction between pulmonary vascular thrombus and the right heart. Depending on the acute clot burden and pre-existing cardiopulmonary status, abrupt increases in afterload may result in a spectrum of right ventricle (RV) changes.

In acute PE, RV dysfunction is the major predictor of mortality, with overt failure responsible for most initial deaths. While prior risk stratification in acute PE was based on the extent of anatomical clot burden, current algorithms now focus on the status of the RV to identify patients at highest risk of early death and to direct management decisions.

As RV failure causes haemodynamic collapse and shock, the initial branchpoint in treatment is the presence of haemodynamic instability. While there is some variation between guidelines, this definition includes cardiac arrest, shock, persistent hypotension (>15 minutes of systolic blood pressure <90 mmHg, or a decrease ≥40 mmHg), and bradycardia. An acute PE that meets one of these criteria is categorised as high-risk (European Society of Cardiology (ESC)) or massive (American Heart Association (AHA)) disease. Moreover, new respiratory insufficiency — primarily considered to be hypoxemia or significant distress — is also included as a feature of massive disease by the AHA.

While not captured in these initial risk stratification algorithms, certain features may suggest a more advanced disease state. Syncope and pre-syncope, for example, are associated with increased rates of RV dysfunction and short-term mortality. Similarly, clot-in-transit, a term describing mobile right heart thrombi reported in 4–18% of PE patients, heralds worse outcomes and requires an aggressive management approach.

The PE Response Team

Given the complex and often nuanced decisions in PE treatment — particularly in haemodynamically unstable disease — many institutions have created PE response teams (PERT) to assist in the evaluation and treatment of unstable PE patients. While variable in composition, these multidisciplinary groups generally consist of cardiologists, pulmonologists, cardiac surgeons, and interventional radiologists, among other specialists. While data on their use is limited, limited data suggests that PERT creation may be associated with better short-term mortality, particularly among intermediate and high-risk patients.

Haemodynamically Unstable Pulmonary Emboli

Initial resuscitation, anticoagulation, and diagnosis

Accounting for 5–8% of all pulmonary emboli, high-risk or massive PE is infrequent but associated with excessive early mortality, reaching up to 65% in patients who present in total haemodynamic collapse. Most deaths in this population occur due to shock within the first 1–2 hours. Initial management of high-risk or massive PE therefore centres on aggressive resuscitation, rapid diagnosis, and definitive therapy.

In acute PE, initial resuscitation should address cardiopulmonary derangements. For hypotension, cautious fluid resuscitation can be trialled — usually as a bolus of 500 mL or less — with guidance from central venous catheter pressure measurements or echocardiographic inferior vena cava appearance, if available. To not further worsen an already-elevated preload, however, the threshold for vasopressor initiation should be low; inotropes may be helpful but may propagate hypotension and arrhythmias. In massive PE, small case series suggest that inhaled vasodilators may offload the RV to improve haemodynamics and oxygenation. Hypoxemia from ventilation-perfusion mismatch can be corrected for goal oxygen saturation (SpO_2) $\geq 90\%$; however, intubation should be deferred until absolutely necessary given the potential further cardiopulmonary deterioration.

While resuscitation is ongoing, simultaneous evaluation should focus on elucidating the cause of haemodynamic instability. While certain risk factors — prolonged immobility, recent orthopaedic surgery, and active malignancy, among others — may raise suspicion of a PE, multiple calculators including the Wells score can objectively assess probability of this disease. In an unstable patient, a series of bedside tests may further support this diagnosis. An electrocardiogram will exclude acute coronary syndrome and arrythmias but may suggest new RV strain, and ultrasound can demonstrate lower extremity deep venous thrombi. The most important bedside test is arguably echocardiography, which may reveal new right-sided enlargement (RV/LV diameter ratio >1.0), dysfunction, or even clot-in-transit while eliminating other causes such as cardiac tamponade and hypovolemia.

In haemodynamically unstable patients with high suspicion of a PE, anticoagulation with unfractionated heparin (UFH) should be started immediately in the absence of contraindications. Compared to low molecular weight heparin (LMWH) and oral anticoagulants, UFH allows for rapid and frequent titration to therapeutic dose, as well as quick reversal. Guidelines generally recommend delivery of an 80 μ/kg intravenous bolus followed by initial infusion at 18 μ/kg/hour to target an activated partial thromboplastin time (aPTT) of 1.5–2.5 times the control range or an anti-Xa level of 0.3–0.7 μ/mL.

After initial resuscitation and bedside evaluation, further management depends on (1) the achievement of haemodynamic stability and (2) the availability of computed tomography (CT) pulmonary angiogram. Whenever possible, patients with high suspicion of PE who stabilise with resuscitation should immediately undergo CT pulmonary angiography (CTPA) to confirm PE diagnosis prior to further therapy. As a last resort, empiric thrombolysis in suspected high-risk or massive PE may be considered if CTPA is not emergently available or if persistent haemodynamic instability precludes transport. In these patients, the decision on definitive treatment should be made on an individualised basis. In select cases, mechanical circulatory support may be an option to allow for stabilisation and further workup.

Definitive Reperfusion Therapy

Definitive treatment of a high-risk or massive PE should be focused on immediate reperfusion followed by anticoagulation. Three reperfusion methods have been established and while systemic thrombolysis is the most commonly used, surgical pulmonary embolectomy and catheter-directed thrombolysis play important roles in select populations.

Systemic thrombolysis

Systemic thrombolytics convert plasminogen into plasmin to rapidly lyse fibrin in clot, resulting in a 30–35% reduction in perfusion defect at 24 hours. With rapid afterload reduction, pulmonary arterial pressures and resistance quickly improve, as does RV function on echocardiographic and invasive assessment. While mortality is difficult to evaluate in this critically ill population, there appears to be a benefit with thrombolysis: in an initial study of eight patients, all four randomised to streptokinase survived but those who received only UFH died, prompting early study termination. Recent meta-analyses have shown similar findings: compared to anticoagulation in unstable PE, systemic thrombolysis was associated with reduced risk of recurrent PE and death, although this therapy was notably underutilised.

Major bleeding is the most serious complication of systemic thrombolysis, with intracranial haemorrhage occurring in up to 1.4–1.7% of patients. As such, all patients with massive or high-risk PE require assessment for contraindications prior to systemic thrombolysis (Table 1).

In the absence of any contraindications, confirmed high-risk or massive PE should be treated with immediate systemic thrombolysis. Patients with an elevated bleeding risk merit careful evaluation: those with absolute contraindications may fare best with an alternative reperfusion strategy; however, the benefit of systemic thrombolysis often outweighs risk in patients with relative contraindications.

In acute PE, the most widely utilised lytic agent is alteplase, a second-generation recombinant tissue plasminogen activator (r-tPA). Compared to the first-generation agents streptokinase and urokinase, the fibrin-specific r-tPAs offer multiple advantages including longer half-life, shorter infusion times, and reduced allergic reactions. Based on the patient's clinical status, alteplase is delivered as a peripheral infusion via one of the two strategies: (1) the typical 100 mg dose over 2 hours or (2) the accelerated dose of 0.6 mg/kg to a maximum 50 mg administered over 15 minutes during cardiac arrest or another extreme situation, with the additional 50 mg given at a later time. The third-generation r-tPAs, reteplase, and tenecteplase are under investigation but are not yet approved by the Food and Drug Administration for use in acute PE.

Table 1. Absolute and relative contraindications to systemic thrombolysis, based on European Society of Cardiology and American Heart Association guidelines.

Absolute	Relative

• Structural central nervous system disease
• Prior intracranial haemorrhage or stroke of unknown origin
• Ischemic stroke in previous 3–6 months
• Active bleeding
• Recent*:
  ○ Major trauma
  ○ Significant closed-head or facial trauma with brain injury or bony fracture
  ○ Brain or spinal canal surgery
  ○ Major surgery (generally within 3 weeks)
• Bleeding diathesis
	• Refractory hypertension (systolic blood pressure >180 mmHg or diastolic blood pressure >110 mmHg)
	• Traumatic or prolonged cardiopulmonary resuscitation
	• Non-compressible puncture site
	• Recent:
	  ○ Internal bleeding (2–4 weeks)
	  ○ Transient ischemic attack (within 6 months)
	• Active:
	  ○ Advanced liver disease
	  ○ Peptic ulcer
	  ○ Diabetic retinopathy
	  ○ Pregnancy
	• Pre-existing anticoagulation use
	• Age >75 years

Note: *Recent non-CNS surgery and minor injuries are not necessarily absolute contraindications to thrombolysis but should be evaluated on a case-by-case basis.

There is no consensus on the coordination of UFH and thrombolysis: given the increased bleeding risk, anticoagulation can be stopped during alteplase infusion — and certainly must be held with first-generation thrombolytics — but should be reinitiated when the PTT falls below the therapeutic level. In the event of severe bleeding, alteplase and anticoagulation should immediately be stopped. While heparin can be reversed with protamine, there is no lytic-specific agent and as such, care is supportive. The aminocaproic and tranexamic acids have been used in case reports.

Surgical pulmonary embolectomy

Surgical pulmonary embolectomy is an effective reperfusion treatment for select patients with massive or high-risk PE. Depending on multiple factors including operator expertise and disease severity, reported mortality with this procedure varies widely from 3.6% to 27%. While never compared to systemic thrombolysis in a randomised controlled trial, retrospective series suggest mortality after embolectomy and systemic thrombolysis is at least equivalent. This is driven at least in part by decreased major bleeding with surgical embolectomy; thrombolysis may also be associated with higher risk of stroke and need for PE re-intervention. Notably, mortality with rescue embolectomy after failed lysis is significantly lower compared to repeat thrombolysis.

In high-risk or massive PE, current indications for pulmonary embolectomy include patients with surgically accessible disease who have (1) contraindications to systemic thrombolysis, (2) failed attempt at systemic or catheter-directed lysis, or (3) shock likely to be fatal before lytics can take effect. Given the high potential for sudden decompensation, it is also widely considered to be treatment of choice for patients with clot-in-transit or paradoxical embolism, regardless of PE severity.

Most often performed on cardiopulmonary bypass, surgical pulmonary embolectomy entails a median sternotomy followed by the opening of the pulmonary arteries with extraction of visible clot down to the peripheral vessels. As the risk of death is highest among those with pre-operative cardiac arrest, prolonged cardiopulmonary resuscitation is a contraindication; however, recent surgery and thrombolysis generally do not preclude surgery.

Catheter-directed therapies

Catheter-directed therapies represent a group of novel alternative reperfusion treatments for select high-risk or massive PE patients. This umbrella term encompasses both low-dose lytic infusion via a pulmonary artery catheter to selectively target thrombus as well as mechanical techniques to remove clot including aspiration and fragmentation; these strategies are often used in concert.

In selected patients with massive or high-risk PE, catheter-directed therapy appears to be effective. Among 594 patients with massive PE — the majority of whom received at least a local lytic infusion — the success rate, as defined by cardiopulmonary improvement in the context of in-hospital survival, was 86.5%, with a low rate of major complications of 2.4%. Additional prospective single-arm studies of catheter-directed thrombolysis (CDT) have also noted improved haemodynamics and RV strain in high- and intermediate-risk PE patients. Bleeding risk with CDT varies widely based on disease severity but falls somewhere in between that of anticoagulation alone and that with systemic thrombolysis.

Differences in outcomes between CDT and other reperfusion techniques are not well characterised. Among intermediate and high-risk PE patients, the cohort referred for CDT appears to be more stable — with less frequent shock and cardiac arrest — than the group who received systemic thrombolysis. Regardless, retrospective data suggest CDT is not consistently associated with better survival compared to systemic thrombolysis. Accounting for pre-operative cardiac arrest, mortality is also similar between CDT and surgical embolectomy in massive PE. Randomised comparison of these two modalities is ongoing.

Current guidelines therefore recommend the use of catheter-directed therapies in high-risk or massive PE with (1) contraindications to thrombolysis or (2) failed systemic thrombolysis. These techniques can also be utilised also in patients who are at high risk of death before the onset of systemic lysis; however, the additional time required for the procedure itself should be considered.

Post-reperfusion anticoagulation

After reperfusion therapy, anticoagulation should be initiated. Post-thrombolysis, UFH is the preferred agent and should be restarted when the aPTT falls under 1.5–2.5 times the therapeutic level. Similarly, UFH should be reinitiated when safe from a surgical perspective after embolectomy. After a period of haemodynamic stability, UFH can be transitioned to an oral agent, with preference for a direct oral anticoagulant (DOAC) over a vitamin K antagonist.

Haemodynamically Stable PE

Completion of risk stratification

Haemodynamically stable pulmonary emboli represent a highly variable disease group, ranging from patients who are asymptomatic with incidentally detected disease to those on the verge of cardiopulmonary collapse. As RV injury has negative implications for outcomes, the presence of RV dysfunction is the major determinant of further risk stratification.

In acute PE, RV dysfunction is defined by a characteristic set of laboratory, and imaging findings. In both AHA and ESC guidelines, elevated troponin is indicative of myocardial injury and reflects higher risk of short-term mortality. Similarly, increases in the BNP and NT-proBNP suggest wall stretch and dilation. On imaging, right-sided dysfunction may be evidenced by RV enlargement (RV/LV diameter ratio >0.9–1.0 in four-chamber or transverse view) on CT chest or echocardiogram. Echocardiography may also reveal systolic dysfunction with depressed tricuspid annular plane systolic excursion <16 mm or McConnell's sign. Additional factors such as clot-in-transit or a patent foramen ovale may also be noted.

A haemodynamically stable PE with RV injury or dysfunction is categorised as intermediate-risk (ESC) or submassive (AHA) disease. Given the wide spectrum of right-sided dysfunction even within this group, ESC guidelines further subdivide patients: those with both laboratory and imaging findings of RV dysfunction are grouped as intermediate-high risk, whereas those with only one positive biomarker are considered to be intermediate-low risk. Haemodynamically stable patients with a normal right ventricle are categorised as low risk.

Given the potential impact of a patient's underlying clinical status on outcomes, ESC guidelines on PE risk stratification also incorporate the use of the full or simplified pulmonary embolism severity index (PESI) scores. These metrics weigh comorbidities and clinical status — including heart rate, blood pressure, and malignancy, among other variables — to predict the risk of mortality at 30 days. A PESI score of ≥III or simplified PESI (sPESI) ≥1 is supportive of higher risk disease, with the caveat that these measures do not replace biomarker assessment: laboratory or imaging evidence of RV strain supersedes a negative PESI or sPESI, such that these presentations are still considered to be intermediate-risk.

Treatment of Haemodynamically Stable PE

Management of the haemodynamically stable PE population is nuanced, particularly in the subset with intermediate-risk or submassive disease. The foundation of haemodynamically stable PE treatment is anticoagulation; however, there has been significant interest in the use of advanced therapies in the intermediate-risk population, largely with mixed results.

Systemic thrombolysis

Given the theoretical benefit of more rapid clot breakdown, there was early interest in the application of systemic thrombolysis to the submassive or intermediate-risk PE. In intermediate-risk PE, lytics rapidly improve RV function, which may translate to early clinical stabilisation. In a randomised controlled trial (RCT) of lytics in submassive PE (MAPPET-3), alteplase was associated with a reduction in the primary outcome of inpatient death or clinical deterioration compared to UFH alone. This finding was primarily driven by less frequent decompensation, although 30-day survival was higher in the alteplase-treated group. An RCT of tenecteplase showed similar findings in intermediate-risk PE (PEITHO): compared to UFH, there was a significant decrease in the endpoint of all-cause mortality and haemodynamic collapse at seven days (2.6% versus 5.6%, $p = 0.02$). Again, this finding was primarily due to reduced risk of haemodynamic deterioration — instead of a survival benefit — and additional meta-analyses have shown variable effects of systemic thrombolysis on mortality in cohorts containing intermediate-risk PE patients.

This potential benefit in early mortality occurs at the expense of a consistent and significant increase in major bleeding, particularly among elderly patients. Furthermore, while long-term data are limited, systemic thrombolysis has not been shown to be associated with improvements in mortality, dyspnoea, functional limitation, or RV dysfunction at three years post-treatment. Systemic thrombolysis is therefore not recommended in intermediate-risk or submassive PE.

Catheter-directed therapies

As CDT offers more focused lysis with mitigated bleeding risk, its use in intermediate-risk or submassive PE has been of significant interest. Compared to anticoagulation alone, CDT is associated with more rapid improvements in haemodynamic derangements and echocardiographic RV dysfunction.

To date, there has been one RCT comparing CDT to anticoagulation in submassive or intermediate-risk PE (ULTIMA). Among 59 PE patients with RV dysfunction, 30 received ultrasound-assisted CDT with reduced-dose tPA (10–20 mg over 15 hours). Compared to UFH alone, CDT was associated with a significant decrease in the primary outcome of echocardiographic RV dilation at 24 hours.

Importantly, the more rapid restoration of RV function does not consistently translate to better long-term outcomes in intermediate-risk or submassive PE. As the follow-up period after the acute PE lengthens, anticoagulation and CDT-treated patients experience similar RV recovery. Similarly, CDT does not improve longer-term dyspnoea, oxygen requirements, or mortality. While thrombus organises over time, more rapid lysis with CDT is also not consistently associated with reduced development of chronic thromboembolic pulmonary hypertension. Further comparison of CDT and anticoagulation in intermediate-risk PE is ongoing in the HI-PEITHO study.

Catheter-directed thrombolysis should therefore be utilised on a case-by-case basis in the intermediate-risk or submassive PE population. Within this cohort, there are likely select patients that derive additional benefit from this intervention; however, further work is needed to define these subgroups and their characteristics.

Anticoagulation

Anticoagulation remains the most important treatment for haemodynamically stable PE. In the absence of contraindications, it should be initiated immediately at diagnosis in the vast majority of low-risk PE patients. Notably, there is ongoing debate over its use in the population with an isolated subsegmental PE and no DVT or risk factors. Patients with low-risk PE should not receive systemic thrombolysis or other advanced interventions. While the early management of intermediate-risk disease is more controversial, anticoagulation is the recommended initial treatment for most of this cohort.

In terms of the optimal agent, UFH is preferred only in patients with high-risk PE or with significant risk of short-term decompensation. Patients with low- or stable intermediate-risk disease should initiate an alternative agent such LMWH, fondaparinux, or a direct oral anticoagulant (DOAC).

Furthermore, the diagnosis of a low or intermediate-risk PE does not warrant hospitalisation. Rather, guidelines suggest that a patient who meets the following criteria can be discharged: (1) is stable without significant cardiopulmonary symptoms, (2) has no contraindications to anticoagulation, and (3) has good compliance with close outpatient follow-up. Those with intermediate-risk disease but a high likelihood of decompensation require admission.

Changes in Clinical Status

An acute PE is not a static diagnosis; rather, its cardiopulmonary effects can fluctuate with time. Albeit an atypical outcome, short-term deterioration does occur. Risk factors for precipitous worsening with include residual deep venous thrombosis, central clot location, hypoxemia, and RV strain, among others.

In patients who deteriorate after starting anticoagulation — even in those who have not developed hypotension — the general recommendation is for systemic thrombolysis in the absence of contraindications, although the data surrounding this suggestion is limited. The definition of deterioration is broad but may include worsening haemodynamics (falling systolic blood pressure or progressive tachycardia), respiratory insufficiency, RV dysfunction, or perfusion. Lysis again occurs at the risk of increased bleeding but it is associated with reduced mortality in the deteriorating population.

Conclusion

Acute PE is a complex and nuanced disease; however, given the potential for high morbidity and mortality, rapid risk stratification and treatment initiation are essential. While anticoagulation is the mainstay of therapy across all severities, immediate reperfusion therapy is an important initial step in haemodynamically unstable disease. As understanding of PE pathophysiology and its relation to outcomes grows, there will likely be a role for more refined subgrouping to direct treatment decisions.

Bibliography

Furfaro, D., Stephens, R.S., Streiff, M.B. *et al.* (2017). Catheter-directed thrombolysis for intermediate-risk pulmonary embolism, *Annals of the American Thoracic Society*, 15(2), pp. 134–144.

Giri, J., Sista, A.K., Weinberg, I. *et al.* (2019). Interventional therapies for acute pulmonary embolism: Current status and principles for the development of novel evidence, *A Scientific Statement From the American Heart Association*, *Circulation*, 140(20), pp. e774–e801.

Kearon, C., Akl, E.A., Ornelas, J. *et al.* (2016). Antithrombotic therapy for VTE disease: CHEST guideline and expert panel report, *Chest*, 149(2), pp. 315–352.

Kucher, N., Boekstegers, P., Müller, O.J. *et al.* (2014). Randomized, controlled trial of ultrasound-assisted catheter-directed thrombolysis for acute intermediate-risk pulmonary embolism, *Circulation*, 129(4), pp. 479–486.

Lee, T., Itagaki, S., Chiang, Y.P. *et al.* (2018). Survival and recurrence after acute pulmonary embolism treated with pulmonary embolectomy or thrombolysis in New York State, 1999 to 2013, *The Journal of Thoracic Cardiovascular Surgery*, 155(3), pp. 1084–1090.

Loyalka, P., Ansari, M.Z., Cheema, F.H. *et al.* (2018). Surgical pulmonary embolectomy and catheter-based therapies for acute pulmonary embolism: A contemporary systematic review, *The Journal of Thoracic Cardiovascular Surgery*, 156(6), pp. 2155–2167.

Meyer, G., Vicaut, E., Danays, T. *et al.* (2014). Fibrinolysis for patients with intermediate-risk pulmonary embolism, *The New England Journal of Medicine*, 370(15), pp. 1402–1411.

Pei, D.T., Liu, J., Yaqoob, M. *et al.* (2019). Meta-analysis of catheter directed ultrasound-assisted thrombolysis in pulmonary embolism, *The American Journal of Cardiology*, 124(9), pp. 1470–1477.

Piazza, G., Hohlfelder, B., Jaff, M.R. *et al.* (2015). A prospective, single-arm, multicenter trial of ultrasound-facilitated, catheter-directed, low-dose fibrinolysis for acute massive and submassive pulmonary embolism: The SEATTLE II Study, *JACC Cardiovascular Intervention*, 8(10), pp. 1382–1392.

Stevens, S.M., Woller, S.C., Baumann Kreuziger, L. *et al.* (2021). Antithrombotic therapy for VTE disease: Second update of the CHEST guideline and expert panel report — Executive summary, *Chest*, 160, pp. 2247–2259.

https://doi.org/10.1142/9781800612778_0005

Chapter 5

Systemic Thrombolysis in Acute Pulmonary Embolism: Dose Considerations in Administration of Thrombolytics

Stella M. Savarimuthu, Inderjit Singh, and Akhil Khosla

Section of Pulmonary, Critical Care, and Sleep Medicine,
Yale School of Medicine, New Haven, CT, USA

Abstract

Acute pulmonary embolism (PE) can cause devastating cardiopulmonary effects, including haemodynamic collapse, respiratory failure, and death. Thrombolytic therapies allow for quick-acting dissolution of clot and have been shown to improve outcomes in high-risk pulmonary embolism. However, thrombolysis carries a substantial risk of major bleed, and should be administered with caution. In select populations, half-dose thrombolysis can be utilised instead, though improved clinical outcomes, such as mortality, have not been demonstrated in large-scale studies. In this chapter, we will review the pharmacology of thrombolysis, rationale behind its use in high-risk pulmonary embolism and cardiac arrest, and consideration of half-dose thrombolysis in populations at risk for major bleeding event.

Introduction

Thrombolytic therapies were developed to allow for quick-acting dissolution of clot and have been shown to improve outcomes in high-risk pulmonary embolism. However, thrombolysis is not a benign therapy, and requires careful evaluation of both its benefits and harms. In this chapter, we will review the pharmacology of thrombolytics, use and dosage considerations, contraindications, and application in various clinical settings.

Pharmacology of Thrombolytics

Fibrinolysis occurs in homeostatic conditions to remove unwanted fibrin thrombi. Native plasminogen activators, including tissue plasminogen activator (tPA) and urokinase plasminogen activator (uPA), are stimulated in the presence of fibrin to convert inactive plasminogen to active plasmin, which then binds to and lyses intravascular fibrin.

Plasminogen activators are administered as a therapeutic to rapidly dissolve major thrombi causing ischaemic injury, as in the case of acute myocardial infarction, cerebral infarction, or pulmonary embolism. When administered in high doses, plasminogen activators promote the generation of excessive plasmin to the point of degrading other coagulation factors (namely, Factors V and VIII) in addition to fibrin, and preventing formation of clot; this explains the risk of bleeding with administration of systemic thrombolysis (ST).

The most common agent used for ST is recombinant tissue-type plasminogen activator (rtPA) such as alteplase, reteplase, or tenecteplase due to its wide availability and ability to be administered rapidly. Alternative agents include streptokinase and recombinant human urokinase, though these are not available in the United States for this indication. The approved dose for intravenous alteplase in acute PE is 100 mg administered as an infusion over 2 hours with or without a bolus of 10–20 mg; cardiac arrest dosing is discussed later in this chapter.

As a comparator, the physiologic concentration of endogenous tPA is typically between 5 and 10 nanograms/mL. tPA is cleared via hepatic metabolism; it has a circulating half-life of approximately 5 minutes. It is important to note that rtPA usually requires reconstitution prior to administration; a skilled pharmacist, nurse, or healthcare practitioner should be present to ensure adequate preparation.

Indications

Systemic thrombolysis is reserved for cases in which PE has caused haemodynamic or clinical compromise, as there is substantial risk of bleeding complications with the administration of lytic agents. The most widely accepted indication for ST is for patients with high-risk or massive PE. High-risk PE is defined as PE causing shock or sustained hypotension (systolic blood pressure <90 mmHg or a decrease in systolic blood pressure by ≥40 mmHg for 15 minutes), need for vasopressors, and/or cardiac arrest. PE should be first confirmed by imaging with computed tomography pulmonary angiography (CTPA), ventilation perfusion scanning, or pulmonary arteriography. The exception to this is in the cohort of patients who are too unstable for confirmatory testing such as those with severe shock or cardiopulmonary arrest, during which imaging may not be feasible. Point-of-care ultrasound findings such as diagnosis of deep vein thrombosis, right ventricular dysfunction, or right-heart thrombi may help confirm a diagnosis of acute PE when there is a high clinical suspicion in a patient with haemodynamic instability.

Current evidence for ST has relied on observational trials or small randomised controlled trials limited by patient crossover, mixed patient populations, and variable uses of thrombolytic agent. Compared to heparin alone, thrombolytic therapy has been shown to improve pulmonary artery pressures, right ventricular function, and pulmonary perfusion, noted over the first several days following therapy. Several meta-analyses have shown improved mortality with thrombolytic therapy, though with increased risk of bleeding; this benefit was noted in patients with massive or high-risk PE. Systemic thrombolysis has also been shown to result in reduced rates of recurrent thromboembolism compared to anticoagulation alone in high-risk PE.

Multidisciplinary discussion with or without a pulmonary embolism response team (PERT) is key, as the decision to pursue systemic or catheter-based thrombolytic therapy is often nuanced and requires multiple care teams to coordinate. PERTs act as multidisciplinary teams that are activated immediately in response to a pulmonary embolism diagnosis, and typically comprised of Pulmonary/Critical Care, Interventional Radiology or Cardiology, and Cardiac/Thoracic Surgery providers. PERTs can aid in the decision-making around pursuing ST or alternative advanced therapies such as catheter-directed therapies, surgical pulmonary embolectomy, and/or mechanical circulatory support.

Risk Stratification and Use of Thrombolysis

The decision to administer ST is a careful assessment balancing the risk of further decompensation from PE and the risk of possible catastrophic bleeding with systemic lytic therapy. Although other forms of definitive treatment for acute PE exist, ST remains widely available across multiple settings, is easy to obtain, and is faster to administer compared to other therapies for acute PE. In stratifying risk of decompensation from PE, patients are typically categorised into high, intermediate, and low risk groups, as described in ESC guidelines (Chapter 3, Figure 1). However, it is important to recognise that risk stratification can be a dynamic process and should not supersede clinical assessment should a patient require more immediate therapy.

High risk

High-risk PE is associated with high morbidity and mortality. Patients considered to be in the high risk PE category include those with significant hypotension, shock, or cardiac arrest. This not only refers to patients who require vasoactive medications to maintain perfusion but also to those who have demonstrated a systolic blood pressure less than 90 mm Hg for longer than 15 minutes or those with a drop in systolic blood pressure of 40 mm Hg or greater.

In a meta-analysis of thrombolysis in patients with acute PE, thrombolysis was associated with a reduced risk of overall mortality (OR: 0.59) compared with anticoagulation alone, though this effect was noted only with inclusion of studies of high-risk PE. Bleeding rates were estimated at approximately 9.9% for major bleed (defined by the International Society of Thrombosis and Haemostasis) and 1.7% for intracranial haemorrhage.

Intermediate risk

Patients in the intermediate risk group are defined as those who have a PE with increased Pulmonary Embolism Severity Index (PESI) or simplified PESI score and evidence of right ventricular strain as measured by echocardiography, CT scan, and/or biomarkers in the absence of hypotension; other high-risk features include new or worsening hypoxemia and clot in transit. Note, that while high clot burden is not consistently defined in the literature and does not always correlate with right ventricular (RV) dysfunction, it is important to determine the burden and location of pulmonary thromboembolism to determine whether alternatives to systemic lysis (i.e., catheter-based therapies) may be used. Patients in this category are typically subgrouped into intermediate-high and intermediate-low groups to distinguish between those who have imaging and biomarker evidence of RV dysfunction (intermediate-high) from those who have one index of RV dysfunction (intermediate-low).

Treatment with ST for patients with intermediate-risk PE remains controversial. In the PEITHO trial, patients with intermediate risk PE were randomised to receive ST (weight-based tenecteplase) plus anticoagulation or placebo with heparin; patients treated with ST had a reduction in composite 7-day mortality or haemodynamic compromise, though patients in the ST group had a higher incidence of major bleeding (11.5% versus 2.4%) and haemorrhagic stroke (2.0% versus 0.2%) compared with patients treated with anticoagulation alone. Outcomes at 3.5 years, including mortality, RV dysfunction, exercise capacity, and development of chronic thromboembolic pulmonary hypertension, were not significantly different between control and intervention groups. Further studies are needed to determine the benefit of ST in intermediate risk PE.

Alternatives to ST are rapidly evolving and include catheter-directed therapies which may be an alternative treatment option that offers a reduced bleeding risk compared to ST in this population. It remains controversial which intermediate risk patients benefit the most from ST or other advanced therapies, and a PERT consultation can help guide decision-making. If catheter directed therapies are not available, ST (potentially at a reduced dose) may be reserved for patients with intermediate-high risk PE and a low bleed risk when there is evidence of or risk of deterioration such as worsening haemodynamics (sustained or worsening tachycardia, acute hypoxemic respiratory failure), or worsening right ventricular function on echocardiography ST should not be administered for clinically stable intermediate risk PE or those with only mild to moderate RV dysfunction.

Low risk

These patients do not have evidence of right ventricular dysfunction or haemodynamic instability and are able to be treated with anticoagulation alone and ST is not recommended.

Right heart thrombi

Optimal treatment for patients with right-heart thrombi (RHT) is unclear and includes anticoagulation alone, ST, catheter or surgical embolectomy. ST has been associated with improved survival in patients with RHT compared to anticoagulation therapy alone. It is reasonable to consider ST in high-risk and intermediate-high risk PE patients with RHT and evidence of RV dysfunction if there are no contraindications to ST and the patient is considered in a low-risk bleeding category. Ideally, these patients would be evaluated within a PERT to determine the optimal treatment plan.

Logistics of Administration

Preparation

Reliable intravenous (IV) access should be obtained, noting central access is not required for administration of thrombolysis. If invasive procedures are necessary such as central line insertion, intra-osseous insertion, and arterial access, it is favoured to complete these procedures while ST is being prepared or after completion of the ST infusion. Administration of ST in the high-risk PE patient should not be delayed for procedures, as delays to ST may be associated with worse outcomes in this cohort. Caution should be exercised with intubation given the risk of hypotension from sedation and positive pressure ventilation with an already compromised right ventricle; therefore, intubation should only be performed when patients are unable to tolerate or failed non-invasive ventilation.

Patients with high-risk PE require ST or other forms of definitive treatment as soon as possible. ST may be more effective in acute clot (within the first 48 hours) but may still provide benefit in patients who have sub-acute clot (after 6–14 days). ST likely does not have an effect on chronic thrombi, or non-thrombotic PE such as fat-embolism, tumour thrombi, or septic emboli.

If a patient is already on anticoagulation, it is reasonable to switch to unfractionated heparin while awaiting a decision regarding use of thrombolysis. Anticoagulation may be discontinued immediately before and during infusion of thrombolytic, though this practice varies across centres. For example, it is common practice in the United States to hold anticoagulation during the ST infusion, while European guidelines recommend continuing anticoagulation during thrombolysis. It is important to note that ST is not contraindicated in patients on alternative anticoagulation (e.g., low molecular weight heparin, direct oral anticoagulant, vitamin K antagonist), and should not be delayed in an acute situation.

During lytic infusion, clinical exam (including neurologic exam), vital signs, and oxygenation should be monitored closely. Bleeding at procedural sites or mucosa may be noted during thrombolytic infusion; in this case, haemodynamics should be monitored, with application of pressure at open sites as needed.

After thrombolysis

Following thrombolysis, heparin may be resumed without a loading dose when the partial thromboplastin time (PTT) is less than twice the upper limit of normal per hospital laboratory reference ranges. Longer acting or oral agents should be avoided in the first 24 hours after lytic therapy, though can be resumed after clinical stability for 24–48 hours.

Improvement with ST generally occurs in the first 2 hours. In up to 8% of patients, thrombolysis fails to improve haemodynamics and/or right ventricular dysfunction. In these patients, discussion with interventional and surgical specialists may be warranted to consider procedural removal of thrombi.

In the event of major bleed

Change in clinical status (including mental status), change in haemodynamics, or substantial bleed should prompt discontinuation of thrombolysis. If there is a change in neurologic status, the infusion should be stopped immediately with follow-up imaging and/or urgent neurologic or neurosurgical consult.

If additional reversal is needed after thrombolysis has been discontinued, patients may receive supportive transfusions with cryoprecipitate and fresh frozen plasma. Protamine can also be administered to reverse the effects of heparin that may have been given. Surgical consultation should be obtained as necessary.

Risks and Contraindications

The major adverse effect associated with ST is bleeding, with an estimated 6% risk of major bleeding and 3% risk of intracranial haemorrhage.

As discussed in a subsequent chapter, identification of absolute and relative contraindications to thrombolysis should be framed within the larger construct of risks and benefits of anticoagulation.

Absolute contraindications to ST are those scenarios in which administration of lytic therapy has a higher likelihood of debility or death from bleed rather than thromboembolism. These scenarios include active bleeding, bleeding diathesis (e.g., thrombocytopenia), history of haemorrhagic stroke, history of non-haemorrhagic stroke within the last 3 months, intracranial malignancy, or history of intracranial or spinal surgery or trauma within the prior 2 months.

Relative contraindications include those clinical scenarios in which lytic therapy poses a higher-than-average risk of bleed, though with uncertain overall risk of debility and death. These include uncontrolled hypertension (with systolic blood pressure >200 mm Hg or diastolic blood pressure >100 mg Hg), history of non-haemorrhagic stroke occurring earlier than 3 months prior, surgery within the prior 10 days, and pregnancy.

The use of antiplatelets is not a contraindication to systemic lysis, though administration of warfarin with an elevated international normalised ratio (INR) of greater than 1.7 is considered a relative contraindication to systemic lysis. It is important to note that the majority of patients presenting with acute PE will have at least one relative contraindication to anticoagulation, underscoring the need for careful clinical assessment of the risk of bleeding versus propagation of clot.

In those patients in whom the risk of bleed is felt to outweigh the potential benefit derived from ST, options include placement of an inferior vena cava filter or procedural removal of clot (catheter or surgical removal), though recognising patients often require intra-procedural anticoagulation with the latter. Evidence regarding safe use of ST in these populations is sparse.

Full versus Reduced Dosing

Full-dose ST, defined as use of alteplase at 100 mg infused over 2 hours, is primarily indicated in high risk or massive PE (shock (requiring vasopressors) or persistent hypotension despite fluid resuscitation) and right-heart thrombi in the absence of absolute and relative contraindications and a low-bleed risk assessment. The use of full-dose ST is associated with risk of bleed as described above, with increased risk in older patients.

In patients with relative contraindications to ST, thrombolytic can be administered at reduced dosage (50 mg of alteplase over 2 hours). Studies have demonstrated improvement in RV strain and pulmonary artery pressures, comparable to full-dose thrombolysis. In the Moderate Pulmonary Embolism Treated with Thrombolysis (MOPETT) trial, patients with moderate/submassive PE (defined by the extent of clot on CTA or ventilation/perfusion scan) were treated either with thrombolysis with lower dose alteplase (<50% standard dose) or anticoagulation alone. Those treated with low-dose alteplase had lower pulmonary systolic pressure, lower rates of echocardiographic evidence of pulmonary hypertension, and comparable bleeding rates compared with those treated with anticoagulation alone. However, this was a small study with a narrow definition of PE and low rates of RV dysfunction, and thus may not be generalisable; additionally, mortality was not significantly different between groups, and it is unclear what clinical benefit may be seen in patients with lower pulmonary pressures.

Clinical Considerations

Cardiac arrest

Pulmonary embolism is estimated to cause up to 9% of out-of-hospital cardiac arrests and roughly 5% of in-hospital cardiac arrest, though it remains an underrecognised cause due to the difficulty associated with attaining diagnostic confirmation. Small-scale studies have shown variable outcomes with rates of return of spontaneous circulation (ROSC), survival to hospital discharge, and short-term mortality when comparing ST and placebo for all-cause cardiac arrest events. Rates of major bleeding (including any intracranial haemorrhage) in patients receiving ST and cardiopulmonary resuscitation (CPR) is relatively low and the risk of major bleeding from thrombolysis is not significantly higher in patients in cardiac arrest. However, it is unclear if early administration of ST has an impact on ROSC or other clinically relevant outcomes for all-cause cardiac arrest events, as large trial data is lacking.

Small studies specifically assessing patients with cardiac arrest secondary to confirmed PE have showed improved rates of ROSC in patients receiving ST compared to no ST. Given that PE is a potentially reversible cause of cardiac arrest, ST should be pursued when PE is confirmed or suspected to be the cause of cardiac arrest as per 2020 American Heart Association (AHA) guidelines. Common dosing may include alteplase 50-milligram bolus over 2 minutes, followed by a repeat 50-milligram dose after 15 minutes if ROSC is not obtained. If ST is administered during CA, resuscitative efforts should be continued for a minimum of 15 minutes.

Neurologic population

Administration of ST is problematic in patients with recent or acute ischaemic stroke due to the risk of haemorrhagic conversion; note PE may also co-occur with acute ischaemic stroke in the setting of paradoxical embolisation, that is, where clot travels from the venous to arterial circulation via an atrial septal defect or patent foramen ovale. In this patient population, catheter-based therapies may be considered, though ST may be considered if haemodynamic decompensation and/or death from PE is imminent.

Conclusion

Pulmonary embolism is a leading cause of morbidity and mortality. Use of systemic thrombolytics has been shown to improve outcomes for those with high-risk and intermediate-high risk PE. Future research is needed to better understand optimal timing of lytic therapy, risk of bleed with lytics in select populations, and situations requiring either full or half-dose lysis.

Bibliography

Kataria, V., Kohman, K., Jensen, R., and Mora, A. (2021). Usefulness of thrombolysis in cardiac arrest secondary to suspected or confirmed pulmonary embolism, *Proceedings (Baylor University Medical Center)*, 34(4), pp. 442–445.

Konstantinides, S.V., Meyer, G., Becattini, C., Bueno, H., Geersing, G.J., Harjola, V.P, Huisman, M.V., Humbert, M., Jennings, C.S., Jiménez, D., Kucher, N., Lang, I.M., Lankeit, M., Lorusso, R., Mazzolai, L., Meneveau, N., Áinle, F.N., Prandoni, P., Pruszczyk, P., Righini, M., Torbicki, A., Belle, and Zamorano, E.V.J.L. (2020). ESC Scientific Document Group, 2019 ESC guidelines for the diagnosis and management of acute pulmonary embolism developed in collaboration with the European Respiratory Society (ERS): The task force for the diagnosis and management of acute pulmonary embolism of the European Society of Cardiology (ESC), *European Heart Journal*, 41(4), pp. 543–603, https://doi.org/10.1093/eurheartj/ehz405.

Meyer, G., Vicaut, E., Danays, T., Agnelli, G., Becattini, C., Beyer-Westendorf, J., Bluhmki, E., Bouvaist, H., Bren-ner, B., Couturaud, F., Dellas, C., Empen, K. *et al*. (2014). For the PEITHO Investigators. Fibrinolysis for patients with intermediate-risk pulmonary embolism, *The New England Journal of Medicine*, 370, pp. 1402–1141.

Rivera-Lebron, B., McDaniel, M., Ahrar, K., Alrifai, A., Dudzinski, D.M., Fanola, C., Blais, D., Janicke, D., Melamed, R., Mohrien, K., Rozycki, E., Ross, C.B., Klein, A.J., Rali, P., Teman, N.R., Yarboro, L., Ichinose, E., Sharma, A.M., Bartos, J.A. Elder, M., Keeling, B., Palevsky, H., Naydenov, S., Sen, P., Amoroso, N., Rodri-guez-Lopez, J.M., Davis, G.A., Rosovsky, R., Rosenfield, K., Kabrhel, C., Horowitz, J., Giri, J.S., Tapson, V., Channick, R., and PERT Consortium (2019). Diagnosis, treatment and follow up of acute pulmonary embo-lism: Consensus practice from the PERT Consortium, *Clinical and Applied Thrombosis/Hemostasis*, 25, pp. 1–16.

https://doi.org/10.1142/9781800612778_0006

Chapter 6

Catheter-Directed Thrombolysis versus Mechanical Thrombolysis: Who to Consider and What to Expect

Narayan Karunanithy[*]**, Simon Padley**[†]**, and Carole Ridge**[†]

[*]*School of Biomedical Engineering & Imaging Science, Faculty of Life Science & Medicine, King's College London, London, UK*

[†]*Department of Radiology, Royal Brompton and Harefield Hospitals, Guy's and St Thomas' NHS Foundation Trust, London, UK*

Abstract

Treatment strategies in acute pulmonary embolism have expanded to include catheter-directed thrombolysis and percutaneous mechanical thromboaspiration. The choice of treatment modality is strongly influenced by, among other factors, the availability of appropriate expertise and a pulmonary embolism response team. A team-based approach ensures uniform care to all patients using multidisciplinary risk stratification and treatment selection. This expert review summarises the key roles of the pulmonary embolism response team, indications for catheter directed treatment, the published literature supporting its use, technical considerations including concomitant extracorporeal membrane oxygenation, and potential complications of such treatments.

Background

The potential treatment strategies in acute pulmonary embolism (PE) have expanded and include anticoagulation, reperfusion techniques that include systemic thrombolysis (ST), catheter-directed thrombolysis (CDT), percutaneous mechanical thromboaspiration (MT), surgical embolectomy, and mechanical right ventricular support that includes extracorporeal membrane oxygenation (ECMO) or right ventricular assist devices (RVAD). Currently there is a lack of robust evidence comparing the treatment strategies. The decision on choice of treatment modality is therefore strongly influenced by the availability of the specialist services. Local PE Response Team (PERT) formation is recommended to agree on a practical algorithm for treatment escalation. This aids the provision of uniform care to all patients, fosters interdisciplinary collaboration through shared clinical decision making, and serves as a single point of contact for referrers. Risk stratification is a key part of the initial triage of patients presenting with acute PE covered elsewhere in more detail. To summarise, the European Society of Cardiology (ESC) classify high risk PE as that associated with hypotension; intermediate-high risk as that associated with both imaging and cardiac biomarker evidence of RV dysfunction without hypotension and intermediate-low risk if associated with either imaging or cardiac biomarker evidence of right ventricular (RV) dysfunction without hypotension. Catheter-directed reperfusion therapies are not recommended in low and intermediate to low-risk PE.

Indications for Interventional Reperfusion Therapy

In high-risk PE, catheter-based reperfusion therapies are considered in the following scenarios:

(1) ST contraindicated due to bleeding risk.
(2) Continued haemodynamic instability despite ST.
(3) Continued RV dysfunction and residual thrombus burden despite ST.

In intermediate-high risk PE, catheter-based reperfusion therapies are considered in:

(1) Patients at increased risk of impending clinical deterioration based on vital signs, severity of RV dysfunction, tissue perfusion, or gas

exchange who have not yet developed hypotension and have a relative/absolute contraindication to ST.

(2) Patients who are "stuck" with persistent RV dysfunction despite 24–48 hours anticoagulation.

Interventional Reperfusion Techniques

Catheter-directed thrombolysis

CDT involves the placement of pulmonary artery catheters under fluoroscopic guidance directly into thrombus in one or both pulmonary arteries followed by infusion of low doses of a thrombolytic drug, typically alteplase, at 1 mg/hour/catheter. CDT may be performed using an infusion device such as a Cragg-McNamara catheter (Medtronic, Tolochenaz, Switzerland) or an ultrasound-assisted infusion catheter, such as the EKOS Endovascular System (Boston Scientific, Voisins-le-Bretonneux, France). The infusion catheter has multiple side holes through which thrombolysis is slowly instilled, but bolus injection of the lytic drug can be performed at the time of insertion (Figure 1). The EKOS device is 5.4 Fr and has the added advantage of a central ultrasonic core which fragments thrombus and disperses the thrombolytic agent. The advantage of the ultrasound-assisted catheter (USAC)-directed approach is the localised administration of thrombolytic drugs in relatively low doses, typically ranging from 4 to 12 mg per lung, with infusion durations of 4–24 hours. This may translate into a lower risk of major bleeding even in those considered high risk. Given the usual infusion duration of several hours, patients needing immediate restoration of haemodynamics may not be ideal candidates for CDT.

The only prospective, randomised controlled trial of this device to date, known as the ULTIMA trial, compared unfractionated heparin (UFH) alone with ultrasound-assisted CDT plus UFH (Kucher *et al.*, 2014, Table 1). The latter group demonstrated improved RV:Left Ventricle (LV) diameter ratio in the first 24 hours, with a very low risk of bleeding. A larger single-arm prospective trial of ultrasound-assisted CDT, known as SEATTLE II, additionally showed early reduction in pulmonary artery pressures and computed tomographic (CT) obstruction index, with a 10% rate of moderate haemorrhagic complications but no events of intracranial haemorrhage (Table 1). The use of low molecular weight heparin

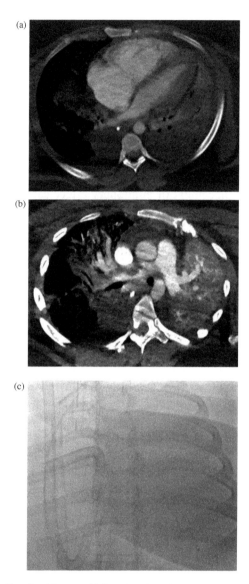

Figure 1. Axial CT of a 26-year-old female with high risk pulmonary embolism on a background of pneumonia. The right-sided chambers and main pulmonary artery (a, b) are dilated and there are bilateral obstructive PE. An RVAD was placed into the right pulmonary artery for immediate reperfusion and subsequently, when only slight improvement was observed, an EKOS catheter was placed in the left lower lobe pulmonary artery where there was persistent vascular occlusion. The striated wire within the catheter represents the ultrasonic core (c).

(LMWH) before and after CDT appears safe, as is subsequent transition to oral anticoagulation.

Mechanical thromboaspiration

This technique involves placing a larger bore catheter than used with CDT into one or both pulmonary arteries with direct aspiration of thrombus allowing immediate restoration of flow. This can be used in combination with CDT. The advantage of MT is that it may be used in patients with high bleeding risk or in those with contraindications to systemic antico-agulation. In the setting of high-risk PE, where rapid restoration of perfusion is preferred to reduce RV end diastolic pressure and offload the RV, MT is considered when the patient has a relative or absolute contraindication to ST. CDT is used as an adjunct in this situation. Additionally, MT is also considered an alternative for surgical embolectomy when the patient has multiple comorbidities.

The Penumbra Indigo system (Penumbra, Berlin, Germany) consists of an 8 Fr single end-hole catheter that aspirates thrombus by combining suction via a pump and a coaxial separator. The latter is a microwire which is intermittently advanced through the end-hole to minimise catheter occlusion and encourage thrombus separation. If the catheter is aspirating in a patent vessel, a phenomenon known as "free flow", post-procedural anaemia may occur due to inadvertent aspiration of non-thrombotic material. This should be minimised by the operator. The most recent iteration of the Penumbra device, the Lightning catheter, offers a 12 Fr system with a free flow sensor. This potentially allows greater aspiration while controlling unintentional blood loss.

EXTRACT-PE (Table 1) is a prospective multicentre single-arm study which describes the Penumbra Indigo catheter's uses and outcomes. The study achieved a significant reduction in RV:LV ratio at 48 hours ($p < 0.0001$) and in 98.3% of cases, this was achieved with no intraprocedural thrombolytic use and very low device-related complications (1.7%).

The FlowTriever (Inari Medical, Basel, Germany) is a large-bore 22 Fr cannula placed into the pulmonary artery to aspirate thrombus with manual suction applied with use of a large aspiration syringe. The FlowTriever device was evaluated in the prospective multicentre single-arm FLARE trial (Table 1). A significant RV:LV ratio reduction at 48 hours was

Table 1.   Reported outcomes for catheter directed therapies for PE.

Author and year	Technique	Inclusion criteria	Device used	Number of patients (n)	Study type	Contrain-dication to ST	Outcomes measured	Improvement in outcome
Sista et al. (2021)	Catheter-directed thrombectomy	Submassive PE	Indigo aspiration catheter	119	Prospective single arm	No	RV/LV ratio	1.47–1.04 ($p < 0.0001$)
Toma et al. (2020)	Thrombectomy	Massive or high risk submassive PE	Inari Flowtriever®	34	Retrospective cohort study	Yes, all patients	(1) Cardiac index (CI) (2) Mean pulmonary artery pressure (MPAP)	(1) From 2.0 ± 0.1 to 2.4 ± 0.1 L/min/m² ($p = 0.01$) (2) From 33.2 ± 1.6 to 25.0 ± 1.5 mmHg ($p = 0.01$)
Wible et al. (2019)	Catheter-directed thrombectomy	Massive and submassive PE	Inari Flowtriever®	46	Retrospective cohort	No	Mean pulmonary artery pressure (MPAP) from baseline to 48 hours	33.9 ± 8.9 to 27.0 ± 9.0 mm Hg ($p < 0.0001$)
Tu et al. (2019)	Catheter-directed thrombectomy	Intermediate Risk PE	Inari Flowtriever®	104	Prospective single arm	No	RV/LV ratio from baseline to 48 hours	1.56–1.15
Mohan et al. (2018)	USAT	Submassive PE	Ekosonic®	30	Retrospective cohort study	No	RV/LV ratio from baseline to 24–48 hours	1.48 ± 0.32 to 1.17 ± 0.26 ($p < 0.001$)
Piazza et al. (2015)	USAT	Massive and Submassive PE	Ekosonic®	149	Prospective single arm	Yes	(1) RV/LV ratio (2) Mean pulmonary artery pressure (MPAP) from baseline to 24–48 hours	(1) 1.55–1.13 ($p < 0.0001$) (2) 51.4 mm Hg to 36.9 mm Hg ($p < 0.0001$)
Kucher et al. (2014)	Ultrasound assisted catheter-directed thrombolysis (USAT) or systemic anticoagulation	Intermediate risk PE	Ekosonic®	59	Randomised controlled trial	No	RV/LV ratio at baseline and 24 hours	1.28 ± 0.19 to 0.99 ± 0.17

achieved. Additionally, 98% patients received no thrombolytic drugs, with 0% device-related complications. Over one-third of studied patients did not require intensive care unit (ICU) admission.

At present, there is lack of evidence providing a randomised comparison of the available interventional treatments to treat high and intermediate-high risk acute PE patients. In addition, there is lack of clarity where the interventional treatment strategies sit beside surgical embolectomy and mechanical haemodynamic support (i.e., ECMO and RVAD). When available, mechanical haemodynamic support can provide immediate stabilisation of high-risk PE, refractory cardiogenic shock, or cardiac arrest (Figure 1), and it can serve as a bridge to the interventional reperfusion techniques described.

Pre- and Peri-Procedural Considerations

Haemodynamic management of high-risk PE includes early vasopressor use (e.g., noradrenaline), cautious volume administration and avoiding preload reduction with diuretics. Intubation and general anaesthesia should be avoided where possible in this patient cohort as the associated reduction in peripheral vascular resistance can prove to be catastrophic. If a haemodynamically unstable patient with PE requires intubation, it is ideally performed by an experienced provider, with vasopressor therapy immediately available, and with the understanding that further haemodynamic deterioration could occur. Mechanical ventilation should focus on avoiding hypercapnia and excessive positive end-expiratory pressure.

Cardiopulmonary resuscitation

The potential for decompensation in the high and intermediate-high risk patient cohorts should always be expected and the catheter lab environment should be equipped with all appropriate resuscitation equipment.

Anticoagulation

Anticoagulation remains the first line treatment for acute PE. The decision to proceed to an interventional reperfusion technique may occur at some time interval after the diagnosis of acute PE is made. Prompt commencement of anticoagulation is recommended to reduce the risk of thrombus propagation leading to further RV decompensation. To achieve therapeutic anticoagulation, LMWH, rather than UFH, is recommended. Most operators would be happy to proceed with any of the interventional reperfusion techniques described with the patient therapeutically anticoagulated.

Procedural technique

Thorough evaluation of the pre-procedure CTPA is essential to appreciate the extent and distribution of the thrombus. The echocardiogram is also reviewed for presence of concomitant right atrial thrombus and patent foramen ovale. This is additional to the routine echocardiographic assessment for evidence of RV dysfunction.

Options for venous access are usually the common femoral or internal jugular veins under ultrasound guidance. The vena cava, right atrium, right ventricle, and pulmonary arteries are crossed under fluoroscopic guidance, ideally initially crossing the heart with a pigtail catheter to avoid papillary muscle injury, followed by over guidewire exchange for the therapeutic catheter once pulmonary arterial position has been achieved. The catheters used for CDT are typically placed in the inferior lobar segmental arteries to facilitate thrombus clearance early in those segments where most of the gas exchange occurs. If MT is performed, a guide sheath should be placed in the ipsilateral pulmonary artery to prevent loss of access and facilitate catheter exchange. The EKOS catheter requires saline infusion through the ultrasonic core during treatment to prevent overheating, and the access sheath patency is maintained with UFH infusion, the latter is also the case with MT. Fibrinogen should be checked at least once daily and replacement with fibrinogen concentrate should be given to maintain fibrinogen >1.5 g/L. Heparin Anti-Xa level should be maintained between 0.3 and 0.7 IU/mL.

Post-procedural considerations

Post-procedural considerations include monitoring for haemorrhage and consideration of the need for further thrombolysis. The majority of patients are monitored in an ICU environment. In the case of CDT, a sheath and catheter will have been sutured to the cutaneous access point upon transfer from the catheter laboratory to ICU. When treatment is discontinued, sheath removal is usually performed at the bedside, followed by manual pressure. A post-procedural haemoglobin drop is an expected observation as a result of MT as blood is also aspirated at the time of clot aspiration to the extent that a drop of 2 g/dL can be expected. Next-day CT or fluoroscopic pulmonary angiography is a useful method to identify patients needing additional therapy including extended CDT and/or mechanical or suction thrombectomy in acute PE management. Perfusion imaging, either with dual energy CT, or perfusion scintigraphy, if available, can provide a quantitative assessment of improvement after catheter directed interventions for PE (Figure 2).

Considerations in the Patient on ECMO

There are a widening range of indications for ECMO, and the availability of the technique is increasing as more centres become capable of delivering this supportive therapy. Patients with high-risk PE and associated circulatory collapse may require urgent haemodynamic stabilisation, including ECMO. Once the patient has been established on ECMO, specific considerations will influence the approach to intervention: e.g. whether to thrombolyse or aspirate clot in the pulmonary artery. Equally, patients who have been established on ECMO as a form of circulatory support for respiratory or cardiac failure, may develop large central thrombosis despite routine anticoagulation utilised for maintenance of ECMO circuit patency. In other circumstances (recent surgery, intracranial haemorrhage), the patient may require ECMO support with minimal anticoagulation.

The configuration of ECMO support can be broadly divided into veno-venous ECMO and veno-arterial ECMO. Access may be central or peripheral, with a femoral vein access from the left and the right sides, for placement of extraction and return cannulas, being the most frequent arrangement. As a result of the presence of an established ECMO circuit, access routes for placement of CDT catheters and for the placement and manipulation of MT catheters may have to be adapted. In general, it will still be possible to place the relevant device from either the femoral or jugular vein, with jugular access being the most utilised approach. When bilateral catheter placement is required, then unilateral or bilateral access can be considered. Unilateral access can be performed using a multilumen sheath in the case of CDT. These patients are quite likely to already be systemically fully anticoagulated

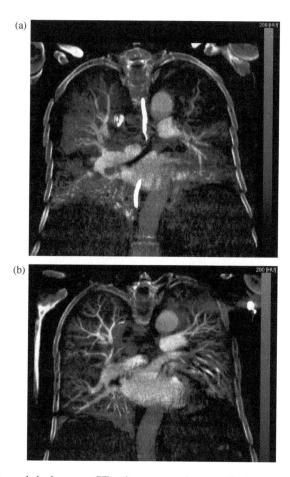

Figure 2. Coronal dual energy CT pulmonary angiogram of a 59-year-old male with COVID pneumonitis and hypotension demonstrates an occlusive filling defect in the left pulmonary artery consistent with an acute pulmonary thrombus, the main pulmonary artery is dilated. The overlaid iodine map demonstrates marked hypo-enhancement of the left lung (a). The patient underwent pulmonary thrombolysis using ultrasound assisted thrombolysis. A coronal iodine map 4 months after thrombolysis and anticoagulant therapy demonstrates improved left pulmonary iodine enhancement (b).

but this is not in itself a barrier to catheter-based intervention. In our practice, combined thrombolysis and heparinisation is closely monitored with Heparin Anti-Xa levels checked every 4 hours after the start of infusion, and the dose is adjusted to keep the Heparin Anti-Xa between 0.3 and 0.5 IU/mL, along with close monitoring of fibrinogen and platelet levels.

Patients may require ECMO support due to single organ failure or multiorgan failure. As a result, the parameters most utilised to monitor the efficacy of therapy in patients where PE is the primary presenting pathology may be less informative. However, pulmonary artery pressures and repeat echo assessment, as well as vasopressor and ECMO support requirements, will allow assessment of clinical evolution. Early repeat CTPA or catheter-based angiography are also typically required in the 24 hours after either CTD of thrombolysis (Figure 2).

Outcomes

Initial data indicate that both CDT and MT are safe, and effective in reducing right ventricular strain in carefully selected patients. Table 1 summarises the findings of key publications, and all reported studies describe either a statistically significant reduction in either RV/LV ratio or estimated mean pulmonary artery pressure. There is however a lack of side-by-side comparison of CDT and thrombectomy approaches, and limited comparative data showing superiority over ST. However, the low reported rates of haemorrhagic complications indicate that catheter-directed intervention for PE are suitable in the case of high and intermediate-high risk PE, particularly for patients who are at high risk of bleeding and death from massive blood loss due to anticoagulant therapy.

Complications

The main complications associated with CDT and MT include major haemorrhage. There are only two reported cases of pulmonary artery injury, and the majority of major haemorrhagic complications arise either from the access site or at other unrelated sites. Procedural mortality due to treatment is low, ranging from 0% to 3% with either CDT or thrombectomy. Table 2 details the reported complications and their incidence in the recent literature. If haemorrhage is suspected during CDT, the infusion should be discontinued with monitoring of Anti-Xa, fibrinogen and platelet levels, and appropriate transfusion. Tighter control of anti-Xa

Table 2.   Reported complications due to catheter-directed interventions for PE.

Author and year	Technique	Number of patients (*n*)	Contrain-dication to ST	Major haemorrhage (*n*)	Pulmonary artery injury	Procedure-related death (*n*, %)	Duration of follow-up (days)
Toma *et al.* (2020)	Thrombectomy	34	Yes	0	0	1, (3)	205
Tu *et al.* (2019)	Catheter-directed thrombectomy	104	No	1	1	0	30
Mohan *et al.* (2018)	USAT	30	No	0	0	0	30
Piazza *et al.* (2015)	USAT	149	Yes	15 (4 at access site)	0	3	30
Kucher *et al.* (2014)	Ultrasound assisted Catheter-directed Thrombolysis	59 (30 underwent USAT)	No	0	0	0 in the USAT group	90
Sista *et al.* (2021)	Catheter-directed thrombectomy	119	No	2	1	1	30
Wible *et al.* (2019)	Catheter-directed thrombectomy	46	No	1	0	0	30

levels with a limit of 0.3 and 0.5 IU/mL should be applied. While pulmonary artery injury is rarely reported as a result of MT, this possibility merits a careful risk assessment of performing centres, ideally with the provision of cardiothoracic surgical support for the procedure.

Summary

Treatment strategies in acute PE have expanded in the past decade to include CDT and MT. The selection of which treatment modality is influenced by the availability of these specialist procedures and requires the assistance of a PERT team to provide uniform care to all patients and share clinical decision-making. Patients with high risk and intermediate-high risk PE should be considered for catheter-directed therapies within specific clinical scenarios, taking into account the risk of haemorrhage from systemic therapies and the presence of haemodynamic instability. While initial data lack side-by-side comparisons to determine superiority,

CDT and MT both appear to offer a safe option for prompt reduction in right ventricular compromise with low reported major complication rates.

Bibliography

Kucher, N., Boekstegers, P., Müller, O.J. *et al.* (2014). Randomized, controlled trial of ultrasound-assisted catheter-directed thrombolysis for acute interme-diate-risk pulmonary embolism, *Circulation*, 129(4), pp. 479–486.

Price, L.C., Garfield, B., Bleakley, C., Keeling, A.G.M., Mcfadyen, C., McCabe, C., Ridge, C.A., Wort, S.J., Price, S., and Arachchillage, D.J. (2020). Rescue therapy with thrombolysis in patients with severe COVID-19-associated acute respiratory distress syndrome, *Pulmonary Circulation*, 10(4), pp. 2045894020973906.

Rivera-Lebron, B., McDaniel, M., Ahrar, K. *et al.* (2019). PERT consortium. Diagnosis, treatment and follow up of acute pulmonary embolism: Consensus practice from the PERT Consortium, *Clinical Applied Thrombosis Hemostasis*, 25, pp. 1076029619853037.

Sista, A.K., Horowitz, J.M., Tapson, V.F., Rosenberg, M., Elder, M.D., Schiro, B.J., Dohad, S., Amoroso, N.E., Dexter, D.J., Loh, C.T., Leung, D.A., Bieneman, B.K., Perkowski, P.E., Chuang, M.L., and Benenati, J.F. (2021). EXTRACTPE investigators. Indigo aspiration system for treatment of pul-monary embolism: Results of the EXTRACT-PE trial, *JACC Cardiovascular Intervention*, 14(3), pp. 319–329.

Toma, C., Khandhar, S., Zalewski, A.M., D'Auria, S.J., Tu, T.M., and Jaber, W.A. (2020). Percutaneous thrombectomy in patients with massive and very high-risk submassive acute pulmonary embolism, *Catheterization and Cardiovascular Intervention*, 96(7), pp. 1465–1470.

Tu, T., Toma, C., Tapson, V.F., Adams, C., Jaber, W.A., Silver, M., Khandhar, S., Amin, R., Weinberg, M., Engelhardt, T., Hunter, M., Holmes, D., Hoots, G., Hamdalla, H., Maholic, R.L., Lilly, S.M., Ouriel, K., and Rosen-field, K. (2019). FLARE investigators. A prospective, single-arm, multicenter trial of catheter-directed mechanical thrombectomy for intermediate-risk acute pul-monary embolism: The FLARE study, *JACC Cardiovascular Interventions*, 12(9), pp. 859–869.

Chapter 7

ECMO Referral and Right Ventricular MCS: When Should These Be Considered?

Benjamin Garfield, Richard Trimlett, and Susanna Price

Royal Brompton and Harefield Hospitals, Guy's and St Thomas' NHS Foundation Trust, London, UK

Abstract

Extracorporeal membrane oxygenation (ECMO) is a form of mechanical support for patients with refractory cardiogenic shock or respiratory failure. Massive pulmonary embolism (PE) with ongoing shock despite maximal medical therapy, including thrombolytics, is an emerging indication for ECMO in a carefully selected group of patients. Veno-arterial (VA)-ECMO provides cardiovascular and respiratory support, can be initiated at the bedside and in the context of cardiac arrest (eCPR). Other forms of right ventricular support such as Oxy-RVADs are available in specialist centres but require fluoroscopy and are less widely used. After stabilisation on ECMO the risks and benefits of treatment with anticoagulation, thrombolysis (systemic and catheter-directed), embolectomy, or aspiration and disruption of clot need to be carefully balanced. Current small case series suggest survival in these patients of up to 70%. Further work is needed to define who will benefit most from this emerging technology.

Background

Massive pulmonary embolism (PE) is a medical emergency character-ised by hypotension due to obstruction of the right ventricular outflow tract or proximal pulmonary artery with clot which leads to hypoxia, right ventricular failure, and eventually, if left untreated, to death. The standard and recommended treatment for massive PE is systemic throm-bolysis which results in clot breakdown, thereby reducing right ventricle (RV) afterload and allowing restoration of transpulmonary blood flow. Sometimes, despite thrombolysis patients have persistent hypotension and RV failure. This may be due to persistent clot burden with or with-out RV stunning and/or myocarditis with an inflammatory infiltrate described. These patients will often need support with inotropes, vaso-pressors, pulmonary vasodilators, and careful fluid management in a critical care environment, with ongoing anticoagulation. In many this will be adequate, however, when end organ hypoperfusion and shock persist, in carefully selected patients, mechanical circulatory support (MCS) with extracorporeal membrane oxygenation (ECMO) may have a role in maintaining organ perfusion while buying time for the RV to recover.

Brief History and Background to ECMO

The idea of oxygenating the blood outside of the body and supporting the vital function of both the heart and lungs dates back as far as the 17th century with Hooke conceptualising an oxygenator and Le Gallois hypothesising that injection of arterial blood directly into an organ might be the first step towards immortality. Through the discovery of heparin in 1916 and further advancement in membrane technology the first success-ful use of an extracorporeal oxygenator was documented in a dog in 1929. Over 20 years later in 1953, cardiac bypass was used successfully for the first time in a human, with the first case of ECMO used for respiratory failure reported in the *New England Journal of Medicine* in 1972. Despite initial disappointing results in adults in clinical trials its use has expanded. Through the H1N1 pandemic of 2009, and now the COVID-19 pandemic of 2020 percutaneous veno-venous ECMO (VV-ECMO) is a well-estab-lished supportive therapy for respiratory failure refractory to standard critical care management.

The basic principle in ECMO is that de-oxygenated blood is drained from a large central vein, passed through a pump and then an oxygenator and returned to the circulation fully oxygenated. There are two main types of percutaneous ECMO: VV-ECMO returns oxygenated blood to the venous circulation providing respiratory support, whereas veno-arterial (VA) ECMO returns oxygenated blood to the arterial circulation providing both respiratory and cardiac support. A third form of percutaneous support relevant to PE includes veno-pulmonary artery ECMO otherwise known as a right ventricular assist device (RVAD) with an oxygenator (oxy-RVAD) which drains blood from the venous circulation and returns it directly into the pulmonary artery. This not only provides respiratory support but also bypasses the right ventricle making this configuration particularly helpful in patients with isolated right ventricular failure seen in PE (Figure 1 (a–c)). The pros and cons of each type of device are outlined in Table 2, later in the chapter.

Pathophysiology of RV Failure in Massive PE

Massive "high-risk" PE defined clinically by systemic hypotension, need for ionotropy, or persistent bradycardia kills up to 21.7 per 100,000 people in the UK per year. Mortality in those with hypotension and RV failure is up to 65%. The thin-walled RV is poorly adapted to sudden increases in afterload and quickly decompensates resulting in RV dilation which, alongside the reduction in transpulmonary blood flow and reduced left ventricular (LV) preload, results in a low cardiac output state. As the RV dilates the septum deviates and impinges on the LV cavity, further reducing LV filling and compromising LV ejection. The subsequent reduction in stroke volume and cardiac output leads to coronary hypoperfusion and global myocardial ischaemia. This ischaemia is further compounded due to increased tension in the RV wall which compromises flow through the right coronary artery. RV dilation also results in tricuspid annular dilatation, resulting in significant increases in tricuspid regurgitation, reducing right ventricular ejection. Hypoxia associated with ventilation–perfusion mismatching increases hypoxic pulmonary vasoconstriction and further increases RV afterload. Taken together these processes set up a vicious cycle resulting in end-organ hypoperfusion, electro-mechanical dissociation, and eventually death. Thrombolysis is the mainstay of treatment for massive PE and results in relief of the RV obstruction reversing this vicious cycle and restoring normal physiology.

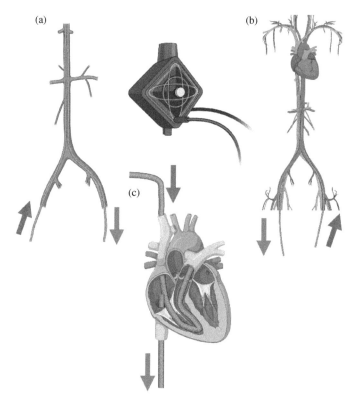

Figure 1.   Graphical illustration of the three main types of ECMO support that might be used in patients with massive PE. These include (a) VV-ECMO, where blood is taken from and returned to the venous system after being pumped through and oxygenator. This provides respiratory but not cardiac support. (b) (VA) ECMO where blood is drained from the venous system and returned to the arterial system. This provides both respiratory and cardiovascular support. Finally, (c) shows an RVAD with and oxygenator where blood is taken from the venous system and pumped through an oxygenator and then through a longer cannula into the pulmonary artery. This supports the right heart and provides oxygenation (image created with BioRender).

Intensive Care Management of Massive PE

While awaiting clot lysis and subsequent restoration of normal physiology, patients may require intensive care support for hypoxia and cardiogenic shock. This requires correction of hypoxia and hypercapnia and careful fluid loading which may be guided by cardiac output monitoring. Excessive over- or under-resuscitation will result in either further dilation or under-filling of the right ventricle leading to a subsequent fall in cardiac output. Vasopressors such as noradrenaline and vasopressin will be required in patients with hypotension to maintain aortic root pressure and right coronary perfusion. Vasopressin may have a theoretical advantage of being more selective for the systemic circulation reducing the potential risk of pulmonary vasoconstriction, although this has not been tested in clinical trials. Inotropes such as dobutamine, milrinone, and in extreme circumstances adrenaline may also have a role in augmenting cardiac output. Inhaled nitric oxide is a selective pulmonary vasodilator that has a potential role in both improving ventilation perfusion matching and off-loading the RV. In the patient with refractory hypoxaemia or shock there may be a role for ECMO as a rescue strategy with small case series demonstrating good outcomes in carefully selected patients.

ECMO for Massive PE

Some current international guidelines on the management of massive PE mention ECMO as a potential intervention in those patients with cardiogenic shock unresponsive to standard therapy; however, there are no current guidelines regarding who should be referred for ECMO and no guidelines regarding which form of ECMO should be implemented.

Suitability and timing

Most patients who require ECMO after a massive PE will need both cardiovascular and respiratory support. VA-ECMO is widely available and can be implemented at the bedside and is therefore, at least in the first instance, the extracorporeal life support (ECLS) support mode of choice in massive PE in most cases (Table 1).

As with all forms of ECLS timing of initiation of ECMO is critical, particularly as too late a referral may result in irreversible multiorgan failure refractory to any form of support. Early cannulation, outside of extracorporeal cardiopulmonary resuscitation (ECPR), should also be avoided as ECMO may not be required if the patient responds favourably to evidenced-based thrombolytic therapy. Young patients at high risk of deterioration in Society for Cardiovascular Angiography and Intervention (SCAI) shock stages B, C, and D might alert clinicians to the future need for ECLS. Early discussion with local services or referral centres is encouraged at this stage particularly if standard therapy with thrombolysis has been unsuccessful in restoring cardiac output and tissue perfusion. The possibility of surgical embolectomy should also be explored but the expertise to perform the technique is normally reserved in a few centres to a few surgeons, limiting its applicability outside of specialist cardiothoracic units. In contrast, mobile ECMO can be initiated in theatre with fluoroscopy or at the bedside. Furthermore, a combined approach with rescue embolectomy in a stable patient established on VA-ECMO may have a survival advantage.

Timing is further complicated in these patients by the inherent risks of bleeding associated with cannulation and the application of prior anticoagulation and thrombolytic therapy. Most thrombolytic agents have a half-life of between 4 and 5 minutes. The anticoagulant effect lasts far longer. The risk of bleeding on cannulation needs to be weighed against the risk of delaying establishment of ECLS and must be determined on a case by case basis.

Table 1. Factors to consider in establishing suitability and timing of ECMO in massive PE.

Diagnosis	Secure diagnosis of PE by CTPA or echocardiography
Treatment	• Failed thrombolysis or thrombolysis contraindicated
	• Unable to immediately attempt surgical embolectomy
	• Cardiac arrest with ongoing resuscitation
Support	• Maximal and optimal medical support on the ICU
Stage of shock	• Patients will be in SCAI C, D, or E cardiogenic shock
	• C — "Classic" low cardiac output state
	• D — "Deteriorating" despite inotropes and vasopressors
	• E — "Extremis" undergoing CPR
Contraindications	• Age and significant comorbidities
	• Inability to match the patients cardiac output needs
	• Vasoplegic or septic shock
	• Futility
	• Duration of no flow in the event of cardiac arrest >5 minutes
	• STOP criteria: (haematological malignancy, significant intracranial bleed, significant CVA, concomitant life-limiting condition, eCPR/prolonged CPR)

Notes: SCAI: Society for Cardiovascular Angiography and Intervention; CPR: cardiopulmonary resuscitation; CVA: cerebrovascular accident.

Referral, retrieval, and cannulation

Patients may need to be cannulated at the referring hospital by a mobile ECMO retrieval team. The model used in our centre includes a retrieval team combining five essential elements: decision-maker, imager, cannulator, transfer specialist, perfusionist, and ECMO nurse specialist. Individuals may have more than one role, and the skill-mix will be adapted according to the individual patient situation (i.e., decision for oxy-RVAD would necessitate interventional cardiologist and fluoroscopic imaging versus VA-ECMO allows bedside cannulation under echo/US guidance by anaesthetist/surgeon/intensivist).

The retrieval team will assess the patient remotely using clinical, laboratory, radiological, and echocardiographic parameters. If the patient is deemed to be suitable and need ECMO the team attends the local hospital and normally performs the cannulation at the bedside under TOE/TTE guidance.

Standard cannulation would be to use a femoral approach, although other options are available, with a 21–25F venous access cannula placed in the femoral vein and advanced cranially into the RA IVC or SVC junction and a 15–17F return cannula placed in the femoral artery. This provides retrograde return of oxygenated blood directly into the aorta bypassing the heart and lungs. Vascular ultrasound is highly recommended particularly for access of the femoral vein in order to avoid significant deep venous clots in an inaccessible vessel.

ECPR is the establishment of VA-ECMO during cardiac arrest to restore the circulation. The criteria for ECPR are outlined in current ELSO guidelines and are similar to those mentioned above in Table 1. Cannulation is described as above and is normally done at the bedside. With the priority being time, guidance is normally provided with trans-thoracic or trans-oesophageal echocardiography in addition to vascular ultrasound.

While the majority of patients with PE will require VA-ECMO, occasionally where carbon dioxide and aggressive ventilation are driving right ventricular dysfunction or there is a concomitant lung pathology VV-ECMO may be indicated. A number of cannulation strategies are possible including bifemoral approach, femoral/jugular venous configuration, and jugular cannulation with a dual lumen catheter.

When established on VA-ECMO further interventions to keep the patient safe are often required. This can be done in a catheter lab in the referring hospital or more commonly in the UK on return to the retrieval unit. A distal reperfusion cannula will be needed to ensure the leg in which the arterial cannula is inserted has adequate distal blood flow. Furthermore, if the patient's heart is not ejecting, which is often the case early in an ECMO run, venting will be required to prevent stasis of blood, thrombus formation and LV distension as the passive diffusion of blood through the right heart fills the left atrium and ventricular and the aortic valve fails to open. This requires one of the three most commonly utilised options either an Impella, intra-aortic balloon pump, or atrial septostomy, all of which not only have their advantages and disadvantages but also significantly add to the complexity of patient care. Our local protocols favour the use of Impella due to its effectiveness in off-loading the ventricle.

In some cases it may be possible to establish the patient on V-PA ECMO with an Oxy-RVAD. This can be the initial form of support or can be a step up from VV-ECMO or a step down from VA-ECMO. This Oxy-RVAD will provide support for the RV, allow oxygenation of blood, potentially disobliterate any persistent thrombus. It also avoids some of the complications of VA-ECMO, including inadequate decompression of the RV.

There are a number of oxy-RVAD cannula available including the Protek DuoTM, a dual lumen catheter taking blood from the RA and putting it back into the RV and a femoral access with a single lumen PA return cannula. There are other forms of RV support that have been used in patients with massive PE. These include Impella RP® System and a number of centrifugal pumps. Some of these systems act without an oxygenator and are therefore less thrombogenic but rely on the patient not being overtly hypoxic which would be unusual in our experience in massive PE. The various forms of support available for the RV with pros and cons of each are detailed in Table 2. Our local preference is to establish VA-ECMO locally and convert to oxy-RVAD if possible.

Ongoing Management of ECMO Support in Patients with Massive PE

A number of strategies are available for managing massive PE after patients are established on ECMO. All have pros and cons and none are evidenced based with studies limited to retrospectively collected data from various cohorts. Furthermore, it is important to remember that ECMO is a support mechanism and treatment of the underlying condition is still required.

Table 2. Advantages and disadvantages of MCS in patients with massive PE.

	Advantages	Disadvantages
VV-ECMO	• Easy venous access • Few ischaemic complications • Low-bleeding (versus VA) • May lower PA pressures by improving oxygenation alone • Low risk from air embolism • Single cannula option available	• Only respiratory support
VA-ECMO	• Peripheral access possible • Cardio-respiratory support • Can provide eCPR • Standardised weaning approaches	• High risk of bleeding • Arterial complications common • Limb ischaemia relatively common • Higher risk from air embolism (i.e., CVA) • May need LV vent
Oxy-RVAD	• Specific RV support • Less bleeding (versus VA ECMO) • Single cannula support • Direct jet of blood into PA may disobliterate thrombus	• Challenging access requires high level of training • Fluoroscopic imaging required • Some configurations splint the RV making weaning studies difficult

Notes: PA: pulmonary artery; eCPR: enhanced cardiopulmonary resuscitation; CVA: cerebrovascular accident; RV: right ventricle.

Anticoagulation and thrombolysis

Anticoagulation alone has been utilised in many patients with PE. VA-ECMO can give time for previously administered thrombolysis to dissolve the clot and for myocardial stunning to resolve. CPR prior to VA-ECMO and the high flows established on oxy-RVAD may dislodge the clot distally or dis-obliterate it. In the largest reported case series on average a third of patients may be managed with anticoagulation alone, with a wide range of variation in local practice between 8% and 52%. Authors have reported both best and worst outcomes in this group but the heterogeneity in the populations studied make this particularly difficult to interpret.

Systemic thrombolysis has been used successfully in patients established on VA-ECMO mainly in the context of ECPR although catheter directed therapy and low dose thrombolysis with endo-vascular ultrasound directed catheters have also been used. These less invasive techniques may be more widely acceptable due to the inherent risks of bleeding with systemic thrombolysis particularly with VA-ECMO. Catheter-directed thrombolysis most of the time with EKOSTM was used in up to 30% of the patients in some studies but was reserved in others to those who were deemed not suitable for surgical embolectomy.

Embolectomy, clot disruption, and aspiration

Surgical embolectomy is an emerging option in patients with massive PE who fail to improve after a few days of ECMO support. Up to 50% of patients in some series have been treated with this modality but as mentioned above the treatment is available in a limited number of centres. According to some studies, there may be some advantage to adopting a surgical strategy combined with VA-ECMO in those who require it. Other options for clot disruption and aspiration are possible with a number of different systems developed recently. Percutaneous mechanical disruption can fragment clot and push it distally relieving obstruction in the proximal pulmonary circulation. Mixed results in case reports with complications including worsening of haemodynamics due to release of vaso-active agents certainly means this technique needs more study before it can be routinely recommended. Percutaneous aspiration devices have also been developed for use in the removal of venous clot. Although case reports of this technology in massive PE have been described, the requirement to steer the catheter into appropriate position has limited its use.

Ongoing monitoring

Once established on ECMO whole body CT is recommended to define the clot burden and rule out complications such as cannula malposition or bleeding.

Patients will need to be anticoagulated for both the ECMO circuit and for their PE and careful monitoring of heparin levels, APTT ratio and ACT is required not only to prevent the circuit from clotting but also to minimise the risk of bleeding.

The circuit health should be monitored by looking at the resistance across the membrane (trans-membrane pressure), the efficiency of oxygen transfer across the membrane (post-oxy arterial blood gas), the clotting factors consumed by the membrane (fibrinogen, platelets and D-dimer), and for signs of haemolysis including but not limited to the plasma free haemoglobin. Changes in any of these parameters and the appearance of fibrin within the circuit should prompt the clinical team to consider changing the circuit.

Careful regular assessment of neurological status is vital for ECMO patients and is especially important after ECPR. The devastating complications of intracranial haemorrhage complicates around 4% of ECMO runs and often leads to significant morbidity and mortality. At an appropriate time, it may be reasonable to wake the patients up and even potentially manage them without mechanical ventilation if their clinical status allows.

As the patient recovers on VA-ECMO if there is concomitant lung disease the mixing cloud where the retrograde flow in the aorta meets the blood ejecting from the heart may be propagated distally in the aorta resulting in hypoxic blood entering the proximal aorta while more distally the blood is well oxygenated giving a falsely high saturation reading. This has been termed "harlequin" syndrome. While this represents the favourable process of myocardial recovery it can also result in deoxygenated blood entering the coronary arteries and the head and neck vessels resulting in myocardial and neurological ischaemia. Monitoring of arterial blood gases and saturations in the right arm should alert clinicians to this process and often requires conversion from VA-ECMO to veno-arterial-venous (VAV-)ECMO where oxygenated blood is returned to both the arterial and venous circulation and may herald a conversion to VV-ECMO. This phenomenon does not occur with the oxy-RVAD which provides oxygenated blood that traverses the lung.

Weaning from ECMO in Massive PE

With clinical and echocardiographic recovery or after embolectomy patients may be able to be weaned from VA-ECMO. A weaning study is done, where ECMO support is gradually reduced for a short period of time to see if the patient can cope off mechanical support and the RV has recovered sufficiently. Weaning from the Oxy-RVAD is complicated by the fact the relatively stiff return cannula that stretches into the PA splints the RV reducing its ability to contract. Expert assessment is needed in this case to ensure the patient is ready for decannulation. A number of strategies have been published for VA-ECMO weaning with our preferred strategy shown in Figure 2.

The venous cannula can normally be removed at the bedside but arterial cannula will often need to be removed in theatre with a closure device or direct arterial repair by a vascular surgeon.

Outcomes of Patients with PE Supported with ECMO

There are no randomised control trials of ECMO support in massive PE. The two largest studies of ECMO support have focussed on respiratory failure, without PE, and quote a survival of between 60% and 70% in carefully selected cohorts. Also, outside of PE, ECPR may improve survival in a cohort of patients with a likely ischaemic aetiology for their cardiac arrest from less than 10% to approximately 50% but can only be provided in selected centres and must be initiated early to be effective,

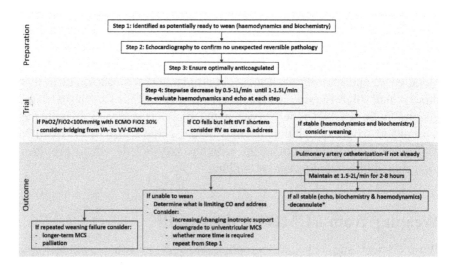

Figure 2. RBH weaning strategy in VA-ECMO. Legend: algorithm for weaning from VA-ECMO in a stepwise manner combining invasive haemodynamic monitoring and advanced echocardiography techniques (adapted from RBH cardiogenic shock handbook with permission).

limiting its widespread applicability. Historical cohort studies suggest that survival in patients with cardiogenic shock supported on VA-ECMO have similar survival of approximately 40–50%.

Patients supported with ECMO for massive PE seem to have slightly better survival than the general VA-ECMO cohorts with those centres performing surgical embolectomy reporting the best outcomes and those patients requiring ECPR having the worst. These have ranged from 40% to over 90% in the short term. RVAD support has also proved successful with survival of up to 90% in some cohorts although again this is based on a small number of case reports limiting the generalisability of these results.

Conclusion

Massive PE is still a major cause of morbidity and mortality. The main cause of death is multiorgan failure due to cardiogenic shock from RV failure. ECMO maybe considered in a group of patients who have cardiogenic shock or hypoxia refractory to standard treatments. VA-ECMO is the main form of ECMO that should be established in PE, however there is a role for VV-ECMO in a minority of patients. Other forms of RV support are available including Oxy-RVADs, which have been used, less frequently but may have a number of advantages. Specialist management of ECMO and PE is needed in expert centres. Protocolised approaches may in the future lead to better outcomes including from ECPR in patients with massive PE.

Bibliography

Al-Bawardy, R., Rosenfield, K., Borges, J., Young, M.N., Albaghdadi, M., Rosovsky, R. *et al.* (2019). Extracorporeal membrane oxygenation in acute massive pulmonary embolism: A case series and review of the literature, *Perfusion*, 34(1), pp. 22–28.

Baran, D.A., Grines, C.L., Bailey, S., Burkhoff, D., Hall, S.A., Henry, T.D. *et al.* (2019). SCAI clinical expert consen-sus statement on the classification of cardiogenic shock: This document was endorsed by the American College of Cardiology (ACC), the American Heart Association (AHA), the Society of Critical Care Medicine (SCCM), and the Society of Thoracic Surgeons (STS) in April 2019, *Catheterization and Cardiovascular Intervention*, 94(1), pp. 29–37.

Bhalla, A. and Attaran, R. (2020). Mechanical circulatory support to treat pulmonary embolism: Venoarterial extracorporeal membrane oxygenation and right ventricular assist devices, *Texas Heart Institute Journal*, 47(3), pp. 202–206.

Corsi, F., Lebreton, G., Brechot, N., Hekimian, G., Nieszkowska, A., Trouillet, J.L. *et al.* (2017). Life-threatening massive pulmonary embolism rescued by venoarterial-extracorporeal membrane oxygenation, *Critical Care*, 21(1), pp. 76.

ELSO (2017). Extracorporeal Life Support Organization (ELSO) general guidelines for all ECLS cases, https://wwwelsoorg/Portals/0/ELSO%20 Guidelines%20General%20All%20ECLS%20Version%201_4pdf.

Ius, F., Hoeper, M.M., Fegbeutel, C., Kuhn, C., Olsson, K., Koigeldiyev, N. *et al.* (2019). Extracorporeal membrane oxygenation and surgical embolectomy for high-risk pulmonary embolism, *European Respiratory Journal*, 53(4), pp. 1801773.

Kapur, N.K., Esposito, M.L., Bader, Y., Morine, K.J., Kiernan, M.S., Pham, D.T. *et al.* (2017). Mechanical circulatory support devices for acute right ventricular failure, *Circulation*, 136(3), pp. 314–326.

Kmiec, L., Philipp, A., Floerchinger, B., Lubnow, M., Unterbuchner, C., Creutzenberg, M. *et al.* (2020). Extracorporeal membrane oxygenation for massive pulmonary embolism as bridge to therapy, *ASAIO Journal*, 6(2), pp. 146–152.

Konstantinides, S.V., Meyer, G., Becattini, C., Bueno, H., Geersing, G.J., Harjola, V.P. *et al.* (2019). ESC Guidelines for the diagnosis and management of acute pulmonary embolism developed in collaboration with the Europe-an Respiratory Society (ERS): The Task Force for the diagnosis and management of acute pulmonary embolism of the European Society of Cardiology (ESC), *European Respiratory Journal*, 54(3), pp. 543–603.

Meneveau, N., Guillon, B., Planquette, B., Piton, G., Kimmoun, A., Gaide-Chevronnay, L. *et al.* (2018). Outcomes after extracorporeal membrane oxygenation for the treatment of high-risk pulmonary embolism: A multicentre series of 52 cases, *European Heart Journal*, 39(47), pp. 4196–4204.

Oh, Y.N., Oh, D.K., Koh, Y., Lim, C.M., Huh, J.W., Lee, J.S. *et al.* (2019). Use of extracorporeal membrane oxygenation in patients with acute high-risk pulmonary embolism: A case series with literature review, *Acute and Critical Care*, 34(2), pp. 148–154.

Pasrija, C., Kronfli, A., George, P., Raithel, M., Boulos, F., Herr, D.L. *et al.* (2018). Utilization of veno-arterial extracorporeal membrane oxygenation for massive pulmonary embolism, *Annals Thoracic Surgery*, 105(2), pp. 498–504.

Part 3

Special Situations

https://doi.org/10.1142/9781800612778_0008

Chapter 8

Acute Pulmonary Embolism with Comorbidities — How Should I Change My Approach?

Chinthaka B. Samaranayake and S. John Wort

Royal Brompton and Harefield Hospitals, Guy's and St Thomas' NHS Foundation Trust, London, UK

Abstract

Management of acute pulmonary embolism (PE) in patients with comorbidities presents several challenges to the treating clinicians and requires careful considerations of risks and benefits associated with anticoagulation, often on a case-by-case basis. Recently, an increasing body of evidence supports the use of direct oral anticoagulants (DOACs) in majority of the patients with PE, although uncertainty about efficacy and safety remains in several patient groups encountered commonly in clinical practice. Duration and dose adjustments of anticoagulation in patients with comorbidities can pose additional challenges to clinicians managing acute PE. This chapter explores the recent developments and latest clinical guidelines in managing acute PE in patients with four broad categories of comorbidities: malignancy, obesity, chronic kidney disease, and thrombocytopenia. Evidence for different classes of anticoagulation, dose adjustments, and durations of therapy are summarised for each group.

Introduction

Acute pulmonary embolism (PE) in patients with comorbidities are associated with increased risk of adverse clinical outcomes, and the management can be challenging. The treating clinicians are often required to balance the risks of treatment, in particular the risk of bleeding, and risk of clinical deterioration and complications from the acute PE. Patients with significant comorbidities are often excluded from clinical trials, therefore high-quality evidence to guide clinical decisions can be limited. This chapter explores some of the challenges of managing acute PE in patients with four broad categories of comorbidities which are commonly encountered in day-to-day clinical practice: malignancy, obesity, chronic kidney disease, and thrombocytopenia.

Malignancy

Malignancy is a hypercoagulable state, with 15–20% of patients developing clinically relevant venous thromboembolism (VTE) during the disease course. Furthermore, treatment of malignancy with chemotherapy, hormone therapy and indwelling central venous access catheters can increase the risk of VTE. Along with symptomatic presentations incidental PEs are also detected on routine staging computed tomography (CT) scans. With improvements in CT scan technology and the introduction of multidetector CT scanners capable of visualisation through to subsegmental level, diagnosis of incidental PE has significantly increased.

Anticoagulation in malignancy-associated PE

Treatment of VTE in patients with malignancy can be challenging due to a three to four-fold increased risk of bleeding complications and recurrence compared to patients without malignancy. In addition, anticoagulation treatment can be complicated by requirement for procedures, comorbidities, and medication interactions.

Subcutaneous low molecular weight heparin (LMWH) has traditionally been considered as the standard treatment for malignancy-associated VTE, except in patients with severe renal impairment, where vitamin K antagonists (VKA) are recommended. Randomised trials have demonstrated superior efficacy of LMWH to VKA in preventing recurrent VTE with similar rates of major bleeding. However, long-term adherence with subcutaneous LMWH is highly variable, ranging from 19% to 70% with higher healthcare costs compared to other anticoagulants.

Direct oral anticoagulants (DOACs) are the preferred first-line anti-coagulation treatment in non-malignancy-associated PE in patients without contraindications. In recent years, five randomised controlled trials have compared the effectiveness and safety of DOACs compared to LMWH in malignancy-associated VTE. All the trials included patients with active cancer diagnosed with acute VTE. Results of individual trials suggest DOACs are non-inferior in rates of recurrent VTE but potentially have higher bleeding rates, particularly in association with luminal gastrointestinal malignancies. Several recent meta-analyses have pooled the currently available evidence, which suggests DOACs are effective in treating cancer-associated VTE with similar, if not better, rates of recurrence at 6 months follow-up. Although head-to-head comparison between different DOACs are not available, a network meta-analysis of the clinical trials showed early evidence to suggest lower rates of bleeding with apixaban in this patient population. Accordingly, guidelines have recommended DOACs as an alternative to LMWH for preventing recurrence in carefully selected patients with malignancy-associated VTE. Caution is recommended in patients with high risk of bleeding, particularly in patients with gastrointestinal and genitourinary cancers.

Asymptomatic incidental PEs in patients with malignancy

Several retrospective studies have indicated that incidental PE in patients with cancer can have important prognostic implications. Furthermore, the rate of recurrent VTE is higher in patients with incidental PE. It is not clear whether the thrombus burden associated with incidental PE influences outcomes. Nevertheless, all clinical guidelines recommend treating incidental PE similarly to symptomatic PE despite the low quality of available evidence. The management of a single asymptomatic sub-segmental PE remains controversial. However, in patients with active cancer or receiving ongoing cancer therapy, the ongoing risk of recurrent VTE would strongly support a decision to initiate anticoagulation therapy, irrespective of the clot burden.

Treatment of PE in patients with primary or metastatic brain tumours

Patients with brain tumours (primary or metastatic) and PE should be offered anticoagulation similarly to other solid organ tumours, unless there are contraindications. There is uncertainty on the best choice of anticoagulation agent due to paucity of randomised trial data in this patient group. Weak evidence suggest possible benefits of a 50% dose reduction of LMWH in patients with intracranial metastases associated with melanoma or renal cell cancer and in patients with brain stem tumours. Additionally, early evidence suggest that DOACs may be associated with lower risk of intracranial haemorrhage compared to LMWH.

Anticoagulation beyond 6 months

Malignancy-associated PE are classified as provoked PEs. In patients who have undergone curative intent cancer treatment with no evidence of active cancer, anticoagulation treatment duration can generally be limited to 6 months. On the other hand, patients with ongoing active malignancy or high risk of recurrence, longer-term anticoagulation should be considered. Continuation of anticoagulation therapy should be based on individual assessment of benefit risk, tolerability, drug availability, and patient preference.

Obesity

Obesity is an independent risk factor for acute VTE. The prothrombotic state associated with obesity is due to multiple factors including immobility, chronic low-grade inflammation, impaired fibrinolysis, increased intra-abdominal pressure, increased fibrinogen, and clotting factor abnormalities. Morbid obesity is associated with increased risk of adverse clinical outcomes following PE and evidence suggest that obese patients have higher rates of recurrent VTE. With increasing prevalence of obesity-associated VTE, addressing management challenges in this patient population has become increasingly relevant.

Management of malignancy associate PE — Summary	
Anticoagulation	• LMWH has traditionally been the recommended treatment in patients without contraindications. • Increasing evidence supports DOACs in treatment of malignancy-associated PE. • DOACs appears to be effective in preventing recurrence with similar rates of major bleeding events compared to LMWH. • Increased rates of major and clinically relevant non-major bleeding are seen in patients with gastrointestinal and genitourinary malignancy with DOACs compared to LMWH.
Incidental PE in malignancy	• Incidental PE should be treated similarly to symptomatic PE.
Treatment of PE in patients with brain tumours	• PE in patients with brain tumours should be offered anticoagulation unless there are contraindications. • Dose reduction strategy can be considered in tumours with high risk of bleeding (e.g., melanoma and renal cell cancer).
Anticoagulation beyond 6 months	• Long-term anticoagulation should be considered in patients with active malignancy or high risk of recurrence.

Choice of anticoagulant for PE in obese patients

Initial anticoagulation

Patients with intermediate or high clinical probability of PE should be initiated on anticoagulation while awaiting diagnostic test results. In routine clinical practice, this is most commonly achieved using LMWH or fondaparinux. Rapid anticoagulant effect can also be achieved with DOACs, with clinical trials showing non-inferior outcomes with first-line treatment with DOACs. However, in the morbidly obese patients unfractionated heparin is recommended for this purpose.

Long-term therapy

Vitamin K antagonists are considered the optimal anticoagulation therapy for PE in morbidly obese patients. The 2016 International Society of Thrombosis and Haemostasis (ISTH) guidelines recommend avoiding

DOACs in individuals with body mass index (BMI) >40 kg/m^2 or a body weight >120 kg, due to lack of robust clinical efficacy data. This has driven concerns about reduced drug exposure and under-dosing of DOACs in morbid obesity. Pharmacokinetic studies have shown that serum peak concentrations of apixaban can be 30% lower and the volume of distribution 24% higher in individuals with high bodyweight compared to reference groups.

More recently, several observational studies have evaluated the "real-world" data on the use of DOACs for treatment of VTE in the obese patient population. A meta-analysis combining this data suggested that DOACs are non-inferior with regard to efficacy and safety compared to warfarin in obesity. Considering the increasing observational evidence in this area, the most recent ISTH guideline statement suggests that the standard dose of rivaroxaban or apixaban are among appropriate anticoagulant options regardless of high BMI and bodyweight. Currently, the guidelines advise against use of dabigatran, edoxaban, or betrixaban for treatment of VTE in obese patients due to the unconvincing data for dabigatran and lack of clinical or pharmacokinetic and pharmacodynamic data for edoxaban and betrixaban. Obtaining serum drug levels for therapeutic monitoring in this population has been suggested; however, testing of DOAC levels is neither widely available nor well validated in real-world clinical settings.

Due to the lack of prospective randomised controlled trials in this area, the recommendations on the use of DOACs in the obese patient population should be considered preliminary. Furthermore, there is significant uncertainty regarding use of DOACs in patients with extremes of weight ((BMI ≥50 kg/m^2 and weight >150 kg), as most studies consider "high weight" as BMI >30 kg/m^2 and weight >120 kg. In addition, each DOAC should be considered individually, rather than grouped as a drug-class.

Dose adjustment of anticoagulants in obese patients

LMWH dosing is weight based and should follow the manufacturers' recommended dosing schedules and recommended maximum daily doses. LMWHs are hydrophilic and mostly remain in the intravascular compartment. In morbidly obese patients with disproportionately more adipose tissue, standard dosing based on actual bodyweight can lead to overdosing and bleeding complications. However, capping the dose at the recommended maximum dose regardless of actual bodyweight may lead to underdosing in extreme obesity. There are no clinical trials examining different dosing strategies in morbidly obese patients and clinical guidelines make varying recommendations. Recent registry-based publications have indicated that an uncapped dosing strategy is associated with significantly higher rates of bleeding complications and capped dosing of LMWH is an acceptable alternative. Therapeutic monitoring with anti-Xa levels is recommended in this patient group. A weight-based dose adjustment is not required with DOACs.

Long-term anticoagulation therapy for obesity-associated PE

Obesity is a risk factor for VTE, and therefore PE in this patient population can be considered as minimally provoked. Unlike most other VTE risk factors, obesity, in the majority of cases, is not a transient risk; therefore, long-term anticoagulation should be considered to reduce the risk of recurrent VTE.

There is robust evidence to suggest reduced dose of DOACs (rivaroxaban 10 mg daily or apixaban 2.5 mg twice daily) are effective in preventing recurrent VTE after 6 months compared to the standard dose in appropriate patients, which is now a widely adopted practice in routine clinical care. However, there are no dedicated analyses or real-world data to support a reduced dose strategy of DOACs in obese patients after initial 6 months for long-term treatment of PE and standard dose should be continued unless there are contraindications.

Treatment of PE following bariatric surgery

Bariatric surgery alters the absorption and bioavailability of many oral drugs due to reduced absorption surfaces, gut transient times, and reduced calorie intake. Apixaban is absorbed throughout the upper gastrointestinal tract, whereas rivaroxaban appears to be absorbed to a significant degree in the stomach requiring ingestion of food for optimal absorption. Dabigatran is absorbed in the proximal small-intestine, whereas edoxaban is dependent on acidic solubility in the stomach. Given the uncertainties in the bioavailability of the DOACs following bariatric surgery, the current recommendation is to initiate parenteral or subcutaneous anticoagulation

Management of PE in obesity — Summary	
Anticoagulation	• Vitamin K antagonists are the recommended anticoagulant agents in morbidly obese patients. • Increasing evidence suggest that DOACs at the standard treatment doses are effective and safe for PE in obesity. • Outside of research settings, DOAC levels are not routinely recommended in this patient population.
Duration of therapy	• Long-term anticoagulation should be considered unless there are other strong transient provoking risk factors for the PE. • In the case of DOACs, standard treatment dose is recommended for long-term treatment due to lack of evidence to support a reduced dose strategy after 6 months of therapy.
Bariatric surgery	• Oral anticoagulation should be avoided following bariatric surgery for at least 4 weeks. • Vitamin K antagonists are commended for longer-term treatment after 4 weeks due to easy access to INR monitoring.

in the early post-operative period. Switching to warfarin can be considered after 4 weeks with close monitoring of the international normalised ratio (INR). DOACs are an alternative option after 4 weeks, however a DOAC trough level is recommended to ensure adequate bioavailability which may not be readily available in most clinical settings.

Chronic Kidney Disease

Chronic kidney disease (CKD) and end-stage renal failure (ESRF) are associated with increased risk of VTE. Several likely mechanisms contributing to the pathogenesis of VTE in CKD have been proposed, including (1) activation of procoagulants such as fibrinogen, factor VII, factor VIII, and von Willebrand factor, (2) decreased endogenous anticoagulants, (3) decreased fibrinolysis, and (4) increased platelet activation and aggregation. Furthermore, patients with nephrotic syndrome have significantly elevated risk of thrombosis due to antithrombin deficiency. Vascular haemodialysis-access related thrombotic events are also commonly encountered in the day-to-day care of patients with ESRF.

Patients with CKD who develop PE have poorer clinical outcomes compared to patients without CKD. Large population-based meta-analyses demonstrate that moderate to severe CKD was associated with increased risk of mortality, VTE recurrence, and major bleeding compared to patients without CKD. These outcomes are likely to be confounded by the presence of other comorbidities in this patient population, however the challenges of PE treatment are also likely to contribute.

Anticoagulation in CKD

Parenteral anticoagulation

Until it is safe to establish on oral anticoagulation, parenteral anticoagulation with unfractionated heparin is recommended in patients with severe renal impairment (creatinine clearance (CrCl) ≤ 30 mL/min).

All LMWHs have a degree of renal clearance and therefore accumulate in the plasma in patients with CKD. Patients with CKD have been excluded from most large randomised control trials performed with LMWHs, and available evidence is based mostly on *post-hoc* analyses and smaller open-label studies. Enoxaparin is licenced for use in renal impairment with a dose reduction (1 mg/kg once daily) for patients with severe renal disease (CrCl < 30 mL/min), and therefore has the largest body of evidence for efficacy and safety in this patient population. However, the safety data on the use of enoxaparin in patients with ESRF is lacking and therefore use in patients with CrCl < 15 mL/min is not recommended. If LMWH is prescribed in patients with CKD, monitoring with anti-Xa levels pre-dose (trough) and 2–4 hours post-dose (peak) before and after the third dose is recommended. Subsequent monitoring should be performed at least twice a week.

Oral anticoagulation

Warfarin has traditionally been the recommended oral anticoagulant in patients with severe CKD and ESRF. Initiation and management of warfarin therapy in patients with CKD can be challenging due to the narrow therapeutic index and multiple drug and food interactions leading to labile INR levels in this patient population. Furthermore, CKD-specific factors need to be considered including warfarin-related nephropathy, warfarin necrosis and vascular calcification. A lower loading dose and slower up-titration is recommended to avoid supratherapeutic anticoagulation levels.

Most recent PE management guidelines recommend avoiding DOACs in patients with severe renal impairment. Dabigatran and to a lesser degree rivaroxaban and apixaban are renally excreted, and therefore drug accumulation in CKD can result in accentuated anticoagulant effects. In large randomised controlled trials on VTE, the dose of dabigatran, rivaroxaban, and apixaban were not reduced in patients with mild–moderate renal dysfunction (CrCl 30–60 mL/min); however, edoxaban was given at a 30 mg dose. Dabigatran is contraindicated in patients with CrCl < 30 mL/min. Rivaroxaban is contraindicated in patients with a CrCl of <15 mL/min and a reduced dose is recommended in those with a CrCl 15–30 mL/min. In patients with CrCl 15–29 mL/min, apixaban should be prescribed at a reduced dose of 2.5 mg twice daily. DOACs should be avoided in patients on renal replacement therapy. Licencing of DOACs in CKD can vary between countries, and therefore local guidelines should be reviewed prior to prescribing.

Management of PE in CKD — Summary	
Parenteral anticoagulation	• Unfractionated heparin is recommended in patients with severe chronic kidney disease (CDK) (creatinine clearance (CrCl) ≤ 30 mL/min).
Oral anticoagulation	• Warfarin is recommended for long-term anticoagulation in severe CKD and end-stage renal failure. • There is increasing evidence supporting efficacy and safety of DOACs at standard treatment doses in mild to moderate CKD (CrCl > 30 mL/min). • Current clinical guidelines recommend against using DOACs in severe renal impairment.

Haematological Conditions

Anticoagulation in thrombocytopenia

Management of acute PE in patients with haematological malignancies and thrombocytopenia can be challenging due to the significant risk of bleeding complications with anticoagulation. Despite the presence of thrombocytopenia, patients with haematological malignancy have a heightened risk of recurrent VTE. There is no robust evidence to instruct management in this patient group and the recommendations in the clinical guidelines are mostly based on expert opinion.

LMWH is currently recommended by all clinical guidelines for initial treatment of PE in patients with thrombocytopenia. However, the optimal dosing regimens in this patient population are unknown. Full dose anticoagulant treatment is generally considered unsafe if platelet count $<50 \times 10^9/L$. Some experts recommend full-dose anticoagulation with platelet transfusion cover if the platelet count is $<50 \times 10^9/L$. However, another approach is the administration of 50% reduced dose LMWH in patients with a platelet count $<50 \times 10^9/L$ and temporarily discontinue anticoagulation with a platelet count $<25 \times 10^9/L$. Use of inferior vena-cava filters may further reduce risk of PE. A recent systematic review could not support one management strategy over another and referring to local institutional practices is recommended. The use of DOACs in the management of PE in patients with thrombocytopenia remains unclear and the recent randomised controlled trials excluded patients with a platelet count $<50 \times 10^9/L$.

Data on the use of anticoagulation in immune mediated thrombocytopenia are lacking; thus, treatment decisions should be made by multidisciplinary teams based on the best available evidence, typically from studies in non-thrombocytopenic patients.

Bibliography

Farge, D., Frere, C., Connors, J.M., Ay, C., Khorana, A.A., Munoz, A. *et al.* (2019). International clinical practice guidelines for the treatment and prophylaxis of venous thromboembolism in patients with cancer, *The Lancet Oncology*, 20, pp. e566–e581.

Key, N.S., Bohlke, K., and Falanga A. (2019). Venous thromboembolism prophylaxis and treatment in patients with cancer: ASCO clinical practice guideline update summary, *Journal of Oncology Practice*, 15, pp. 661–664.

Konstantinides, S.V., Meyer, G., Becattini, C., Bueno, H., Geersing, G.J., Harjola, V.P. *et al.* (2019). ESC Guidelines for the diagnosis and management of acute pulmonary embolism developed in collaboration with the European Respiratory Society (ERS): The Task Force for the diagnosis and management of acute pulmonary embolism of the European Society of Cardiology (ESC), *European Respiratory Journal*, 54(3), pp. 543–603.

Martin, K.A., Beyer-Westendorf, J., Davidson, B.L., Huisman, M.V., Sandset, P.M., and Moll, S. (2021). Use of direct oral anticoagulants in patients with obesity for treatment and prevention of venous thromboembolism: Updated communication from the ISTH SSC Subcommittee on Control of Anticoagulation, *Journal of Thrombosis and Haemostasis*, 19, pp. 1874–1882.

Chapter 9

Acute Pulmonary Embolism with Right Heart Thrombus — Does a Patent Foramen Ovale Matter?

Andrew Constantine and Aleksander Kempny

Department of Cardiology, Royal Brompton and Harefield Hospitals, Guy's and St Thomas' NHS Foundation Trust, London, UK

Abstract

This chapter covers the epidemiology, pathophysiology, diagnosis, and management of two special circumstances in pulmonary embolism care: the presence of right heart thrombus and patent foramen ovale (PFO). Right heart thrombus complicates around 4% of cases of acute pulmonary embolism (PE) and is more common in the presence of haemodynamic instability, larger emboli, and right ventricular dysfunction, whereas PFO is present at the same rate as the general population and usually has little bearing on diagnosis and management of PE, except in rare circumstances. In cases of PE with right heart thrombus, the passage of thrombotic material through the PFO has been documented rarely and can cause paradoxical embolism. A high index of suspicion and multimodality imaging approach are required for diagnosis. International guidelines do not give recommendations for the management of right heart thrombus and PFO in acute PE. Systemic thrombolysis or catheter-directed therapy is typically reserved for patients with haemodynamic instability.

Acute Pulmonary Embolism with Right Heart Thrombus

Epidemiology and pathophysiology

Central thrombi occurring in the context of acute pulmonary embolism (PE) may be detected in the vena cavae, right atrium, right ventricle (RV) or crossing a patent foramen ovale (PFO, see the following section). Right heart thrombus (RHTh) can embolise from the peripheral venous system (thromboembolus) or have formed *in situ* (thrombus).

Morphologically, three types of RHTh exist:

- **Type A:** Long, thin, serpiginous, highly mobile thromboemboli thought to arise from the peripheral veins.
- **Type B:** Non-specific thrombi resembling left ventricular thrombi and usually arising *in situ*. PE may complicate up to 40% of type B thrombus, but is rarely fatal.
- **Type C:** Intermediate characteristics between A and B. May resemble cardiac myxoma, rare.

Type A RHTh is the most common type accompanying deep vein thrombosis and PE. Overall, RHTh are present in around 4% of unselected patients with acute PE, with the exact prevalence and ascertainment rate varying with the severity of the presentation and availability of early echocardiography. In high-risk PE, i.e., PE complicated by cardiac arrest, obstructive shock, or persistent hypotension, where routine early screening echocardiography is available, RHTh are detected in up to 1 in 6 patients. A similarly high rate is found in autopsy studies following fatal PE. This compares to RHTh detectable in 1 in 26 patients with intermediate-risk disease and 1 in 350 patients with low-risk disease. However, in clinical practice, RHTh are rarely visualised, which may be in part because of the lack of availability or utilisation of echocardiography in the acute setting. Alongside PE severity, additional risk factors for the development of RHTh include the presence of RV dysfunction, younger age, previous bleeding, congestive heart failure, cancer, syncope, and oxygen saturation <90%.

It is believed that most RHTh are thromboemboli in transit from the deep veins to the lung. One putative mechanism for the higher rate of RHTh identified in the setting of high-risk PE is that the acutely raised pulmonary vascular resistance and reduced cardiac output increase the transit time of blood through the right heart and promote stasis in the right-sided chambers. Additionally, larger pulmonary emboli causing a more severe clinical picture are likely to be associated with a higher burden of thrombus travelling to the lung. RV dysfunction contributes to a slower transit time and can also promote *in situ* thrombosis.

Diagnosis

RHTh may be diagnosed on one of the several imaging modalities (Table 1). CT pulmonary angiography is the imaging modality of choice to make a diagnosis in patients with suspected PE and may diagnose RHTh as an incidental finding. Suspected cases should be confirmed on echocardiography as incomplete opacification of right heart structure can lead to false positive diagnoses.

Bedside transthoracic echocardiography can identify RHTh with good sensitivity and specificity in addition to providing a comprehensive assessment of RV function. Early transthoracic echocardiography is now a guideline-recommended tool for the diagnostic assessment of patients with haemodynamic instability. In severely ill patients with acute haemodynamic decompensation, echocardiographic evidence of new-onset RV dysfunction can provide sufficient evidence for urgent reperfusion. Visualisation of mobile RHTh during the assessment of a patient with suspected PE strengthens the diagnosis of PE and the decision to treat early. In patients with low-risk acute PE, echocardiography is not recommended as part of the routine diagnostic work-up, but guidelines do advise imaging to exclude RHTh or RV dysfunction if early discharge (within 48 hours of diagnosis) is planned. Validation of this strategy is awaited in future prospective cohort studies.

Transoesophageal echocardiography is not commonly performed in acute PE, but is widely available in certain settings, e.g., in intensive care, and can allow direct visualisation of thromboemboli in the right heart as well as in the main pulmonary artery and proximal branches, with greater accuracy than non-contrast transthoracic echocardiography.

In cases where non-contrast transthoracic echocardiography does not diagnose RHTh despite a high degree of suspicion, contrast echocardiography utilising microsphere intravenous contrast can assist by enhancing the blood pool–myocardial interface, improving endocardial definition

Table 1. Comparison of imaging modalities used in acute PE to detect right heart thrombi/thromboemboli.

Imaging modality	Features of RHTh	Diagnostic sensitivity/ specificity*	Additional benefits	Limitations
Transthoracic echocardiography	Echo-bright structure distinguishable from surrounding anatomical structures, sometimes mobile.	23% ± 12% 96% ± 3.6%	Widely available, portable, and inexpensive. Limited echocardiography possible in cardiac arrest.	Little/no tissue differentiation. May miss small or mural thrombus. Requires good echocardiographic windows.
Contrast echocardiography	Echo-dark structure distinguishable from surrounding anatomical structures, sometimes mobile.	—	Widely available, portable, and inexpensive. Improved endocardial border definition and RV cavity visualisation compared to non-contrast echocardiography.	Cannot differentiate between different intra-cardiac masses.
Transoesophageal echocardiography	As per transthoracic echocardiography.	40% ± 14% 96% ± 3.6%	As per transthoracic echocardiography. Can be performed in patients with poor transthoracic windows, e.g., ventilated patients, and intra-operatively.	Sedation or general anaesthesia carry risks in patients with PE. Better for detection of atrial than ventricular thrombus.
CT pulmonary angiography	Filling defect in the right heart chambers.	—	Guideline recommended test for the confirmation of PE, widely available and relatively inexpensive.	Cannot be used as a confirmatory test.
Contrast-enhanced cardiac MRI	High signal intensity on T1-weighted and T2-weighted images, low intensity on T1-weighted fat saturation images (recent thrombus). Low signal intensity on T1-weighted, T1-weighted fat saturation and T2-weighted images (established thrombus). No uptake of contrast on early or late gadolinium enhancement.	88% ± 9% 99% ± 2%	Allows tissue characterisation, non-operator dependent.	Cannot be performed in haemodynamically unstable patients, relatively expensive and not widely available.

Notes: *Sensitivity and specificity available for left ventricular thrombus.
CT: computed tomography; MRI: myocardial resonance imaging; RHTh: right heart thrombus/thromboembolus.

and increasing the detection rate of intra-cardiac thrombus. Contrast-enhanced echocardiography is an attractive option in patients with acute PE and suspected RHTh as it is non-invasive, cheap, widely available and can be performed in patients who are symptomatic.

Gadolinium contrast-enhanced MRI may detect intracardiac thrombus with a superior sensitivity and specificity to echocardiography and should be considered for stable patients in whom the diagnosis is suspected but has not been diagnosed on echocardiography. Additionally, MRI allows tissue characterisation and differentiation of RHTh from intra-cardiac tumours and anatomical structures, such as prominent Chiari network or persistent Eustachian or Thebesian valves.

Implications for management

Is thrombolysis indicated in patients with acute PE where RHTh has been detected? This is a natural clinical question to ask, especially when visualising thrombotic material in the right-sided chambers, which can be of considerable size. There are currently no evidence-based guidelines for the treatment of acute PE complicated by RHTh; in the absence of randomised controlled trial data and conflicting results from observational studies, international guidelines currently base the need for reperfusion treatment, including thrombolysis, on the presence of haemodynamic instability (high-risk PE). The presence or absence of RHTh is not an indication for reperfusion treatment. It is notable, however, that observational studies of acute PE show that patients with RHTh are more likely to be treated with thrombolysis, even if in the intermediate-risk PE group, despite current guidance. This may be due to the concern about impending embolisation to the lung of thromboembolic material in the heart, leading to a more aggressive management approach in these patients.

The role of thrombophilia screening, prolonged anticoagulation, and vena cava filters in patients with RHTh has not been clarified in trials to date.

Prognostic significance

The presence of RHTh in the setting of acute PE has been associated with increased mortality, but its role as an independent predictor of mortality is still debated. The question remains as to whether the presence of RHTh itself is responsible for the worse outcome in patients with acute PE or if it is a marker for the presence of haemodynamic instability.

In a 2017 meta-analysis of six cohorts that included 15,200 patients with acute symptomatic PE, patients with detectable RHTh had a three-fold increased risk of short-term mortality compared to patients without RHTh (16.7 versus 4.4%). The risk of both all-cause and PE-related mortality was increased in the presence of RHTh, although coexisting RHTh in normotensive patients with PE was not related to a higher all-cause mortality. The presence of RHTh has also been related to an increased risk of PE recurrence. Unlike the finding of large pulmonary arterial thrombi, however, RHTh are not considered a risk factor for the development of chronic thromboembolic disease after acute PE.

Acute PE with Patent Foramen Ovale

Epidemiology, pathophysiology, and diagnosis

In fetal life, the foramen ovale (Latin for "oval hole") is widely patent, allowing oxygenated blood to pass from the right to the left atrium, bypassing the pulmonary vasculature. A PFO is a persistence, after 6–8 weeks of age, of the separation between the septum primum and septum secundum in the anteroseptal portion of the atrial septum (Figure 1). A PFO does not represent a true deficiency of atrial septal tissue and is therefore not considered to be a congenital heart defect. The structure of a PFO is most often a tunnel-like, flap valve that causes intermittent right-to-left shunting when the right atrial pressure surpasses left atrial pressure. In some cases, the septum primum is aneurysmal or the PFO has been "stretched" secondary to right atrial dilatation and remodelling, leading to an elliptical opening between the atria, which can be accompanied by right-to-left or left-to-right shunting depending on the relative differences in right and left atrial pressure.

PFOs are exceptionally common, occurring in around one-quarter of the general adult population. The vast majority of PFOs cause no symptoms and do not require treatment. Rarely, however, a PFO can increase the risk of stroke, particularly in people <55 years old in the setting of an associated condition, such as venous thromboembolism. The prevalence of PFO in the setting of an acute PE is similar to the rate in the general population. In most cases of acute PE, the presence of a PFO has little bearing on the diagnosis, management, or prognosis. Indeed, international

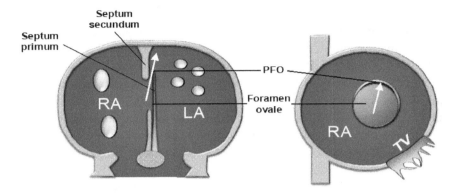

Figure 1.   Patent foramen ovale.

Notes: Schematic diagram of PFO visualised as a separation between the septum primum and septum secundum in the anteroseptal portion of the atrial septum, allowing intermittent right-left shunting (arrow) when the right atrial (RA) pressure surpasses the left atrial (LA) pressure. TV: tricuspid valve. Two circular shapes in RA represent ostium of the inferior and superior vena cava, while circular shapes in LA represent ostia of pulmonary veins.

guidelines do not recommend screening for a PFO in patients presenting with acute PE. In cases complicated by refractory hypoxaemia or paradoxical embolism, however, investigation of a PFO should be undertaken.

A PFO may be visualised during echocardiography, e.g., for assessment of RV function. A PFO may appear as a flash on colour flow Doppler imaging, best visualised in the subcostal four-chamber view on transthoracic echocardiography, or in the bicaval view on transoesophageal echocardiography. However, shunting across a PFO is usually intermittent and may not be detected by standard echocardiography. Confirmation of diagnosis usually requires contrast echocardiography (so-called "bubble study") combined with a Valsalva manoeuvre, with microbubbles that are echogenic and too large to pass through the pulmonary vascular bed. Microbubbles are generated by agitation of fluid (crystalloid, colloid, or a fluid-blood mixture) and 0.5–1 mL of air, injected rapidly into a wide bore cannula in the (right) antecubital vein combined with a Valsalva manoeuvre to transiently augment the right atrial pressure. A long clip length is acquired during injection, in the four-chamber view on transthoracic imaging or bicaval view or similar on transoesophageal echocardiography. Appearance of microbubbles within 3–6 beats after opacification of the right atrium is considered a positive study for the presence of an intra-cardiac shunt. Intrapulmonary shunting, e.g., via a pulmonary arterio-venous malformation, permits the passage of contrast into the left atrium after 3–6 beats. Multiple injections with physiological manoeuvres increase the accuracy of the test. There are no widely accepted universal guidelines for the grading of PFO size, but commonly used criteria are presented in Table 2, along with causes of false-negative and false-positive results. In patients with a negative transthoracic study, but a high degree of suspicion of PFO, a "bubble" study using transoesophageal echocardiography offers better sensitivity and specificity. Biplane imaging can also improve the detection of small shunts. Transcranial Doppler can be used as an alternative or in addition to cardiac imaging to detect microbubbles in the cerebral circulation for the identification of both intracardiac and extracardiac shunts.

Rarely, the interatrial communication is due to congenital heart disease, e.g., an atrial septal defect (ASD). Most commonly, the ASD is of

Table 2. Contrast echocardiography ("bubble study") for diagnosis of PFO: Grading of shunt and causes of false negative and false positive results.

Grading of shunt size	Causes of false negative study
• **Small:** 3–9 contrast bubbles in LA • **Moderate:** 10–30 bubbles • **Large:** >30 bubbles present in the LA	• Inadequate opacification of the RA • Inadequate Valsalva manoeuvre failing to cause an adequate increase RA pressure • Prominent eustachian apparatus causing streaming of blood from the IVC to the inter-atrial septum so that blood reaching the RA from the SVC does not cross the inter-atrial septum • Raised LA pressure, e.g., due to left ventricular diastolic dysfunction or mitral stenosis, causing failure of the RA to increase above the left atrium • Poor imaging quality
	Causes of false positive study
	• Use of incorrect contrast agent • Presence of another form of intra-cardiac (within 3–6 beats) or pulmonary shunt (after 3–6 beats) can be misdiagnosed as a PFO

IVC: inferior vena cava, LA: left atrium; RA: right atrium, and SVC: superior vena cava.

the secundum type, but rarer types exist, including primum ASDs and superior/inferior sinus venosus defects. In the case of a suspected inferior sinus venosus defect, the bubble study should be conducted with agitated saline contract injected via the femoral vein, as streaming of blood from the superior vena cava towards the tricuspid valve may lead to a false negative bubble study following an upper limb injection, also in PFO patients. Similarly, where a persistent left superior vena cava draining into the coronary sinus is suspected, injection into a left antecubital vein may be needed.

Paradoxical embolism: Definition, mechanisms, and implications for management

Paradoxical embolism, first described by Cohnheim in 1877, is the occurrence of arterial thromboembolism originating in the systemic veins or right side of the heart, traversing right-to-left through an intracardiac or pulmonary shunt into the systemic circulation. This can disrupt the blood supply and result in organ or limb ischaemia and/or infarction, presenting with localising features, including the following:

- focal neurological deficit from ischaemic stroke;
- chest pain with ECG changes and regional wall motion abnormalities from myocardial infarction;
- abdominal pain indicating gut ischaemia/infarction;
- loin pain and haematuria resulting from renal infarction;
- a cold and pulseless limb from peripheral arterial occlusion.

Alternatively, the result may be silent infarction, usually identified on axial imaging. The wide range of possible complications, and therefore symptoms, arising from paradoxical embolism presents a diagnostic challenge, and definitive diagnosis essentially requires the detection of a right atrial thrombus straddling the PFO. In clinical practice, this is rarely possible, and diagnosis is circumstantial based on a triad of the following:

1. venous thromboembolism (deep vein thrombosis or PE);
2. an intracardiac (or pulmonary) right-to-left shunt, most frequently a PFO in the context of raised right atrial pressure;

3. systemic arterial thromboembolism, in the absence of other causes, e.g., atrial fibrillation, left ventricular thrombus, or atherosclerotic disease of the thoracic aorta.

Paradoxical embolism is a feared complication of acute PE in the presence of a PFO. Transient right-to-left shunt through a PFO can occur in the presence of normal right heart haemodynamics, the impact of a PE on the right heart may further promote passage of thrombus from the venous to the systemic circulation: If a PE occludes blood flow to a substantial portion of the pulmonary vascular bed, this will cause an acute rise in pulmonary vascular resistance and RV afterload. The pressure load on the right ventricle can lead to ventricular dysfunction in a subset of patients, raising right-sided filling pressures. A right atrial pressure that is greater than left atrial pressure drives right-to-left shunting. Indeed, several case studies have documented thrombi in transit across a PFO associated with systemic thromboembolism. The source of the thrombus is usually the same as that causing the PE, the peripheral deep veins, but there is also a theoretical risk of iatrogenic thrombus as a complication of catheter-directed therapies.

Diffusion-weighted brain MRI has demonstrated silent (or subclinical) multifocal ischaemic lesions in as many as one-third of patients with a PFO after acute PE with RV dysfunction, which are not visible in patients without a PFO. The rates of clinically manifest, acute ischaemic stroke are lower in this setting.

Acute PE and PFO as a Cause of Severe Hypoxaemia

Right-to-left shunting through a PFO (or an ASD) can also lead to severe hypoxaemia in the context of acute PE. Indeed, hypoxaemia is a feature of severe PE, due to the reduction in lung perfusion and increase in dead space ventilation, which results in ventilation–perfusion mismatch in the affected lung segment(s). A co-existing right-to-left shunt would contribute blood to the systemic arterial circulation with the oxygen content of mixed venous blood. Since the shunt bypasses alveolar gas exchange, increasing the fraction of inspired oxygen will not significantly impact the partial pressure of arterial oxygen (except possibly by increasing the mixed venous oxygen content) in the presence of a significant right-to-left shunt. The size of the shunt or shunt ratio (Q_s/Q_t) can be calculated using blood gases from the Berggren equation (or the "shunt equation") with the patient breathing 100% oxygen

$$\frac{Q_s}{Q_t} = \frac{Cc_{O_2} - Ca_{O_2}}{Cc_{O_2} - Cv_{O_2}}$$

Q_s is the shunt flow in litres per minute and Q_t is the total cardiac output. Ca_{O_2} and Cv_{O_2} correspond to the oxygen content of the systemic arterial and mixed venous blood, respectively, and Cc_{O_2} is the oxygen content of the end-capillary blood (taken as equal to the alveolar partial pressure of oxygen).

Hypoxaemia or cyanosis refractory to oxygen supplementation in acute PE should therefore prompt the search for a PFO (or other forms of intra-cardiac or extra-cardiac shunt). Pulmonary reperfusion will usually correct hypoxaemia in this setting.

Acute PE and PFO: Implications for Management

Guidelines on the diagnosis and management of acute PE set their recommendations for anticoagulation, systemic thrombolysis or catheter-directed therapy based on the clinical severity of the PE, regardless of the presence of a PFO. The presence of a PFO, especially with a right-to-left shunt in the context of acute PE, does raise concerns when certain therapies are considered:

- Systemic thrombolysis is contraindicated in patients with acute PE and PFO complicated by paradoxical embolism and clinical stroke, due to the high risk of brain haemorrhage. The risk in the presence of small subclinical brain infarcts is less clear. In both situations, management should involve an acute stroke team.
- Percutaneous catheter-directed treatment, including low-dose *in situ* thrombolysis and mechanical or ultrasound fragmentation of thrombus, involves manipulating a catheter in the right heart chambers. This carries a theoretical risk of catheter-derived thrombus causing a paradoxical embolism, but the safe use of catheter-directed therapy in the presence of a PFO has been reported in case reports and series.

Currently, there is a lack of registry or trial evidence to quantify these risks and inform recommendations regarding modifications of therapy in patients with PE and PFO.

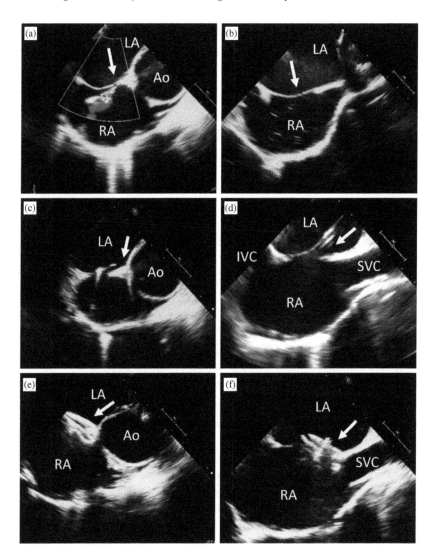

Figure 2.   Transoesophageal echocardiography and percutaneous closure of PFO.

Notes: Transoesophageal echocardiography (TOE) assessment of PFO in aortic (a, c, e) and bicaval (b, d, f) view, before (a–d) and after (e, f) PFO closure using a 25 mm Amplatzer PFO occluder. On 2D imaging, PFO tunnel is often not visible (a and b arrows), but colour Doppler assessment usually reveals a shunt (a, colour jet). During percutaneous PFO closure, a wire and then sheath is inserted through the right atrium (RA) to the left atrium (LA), demonstrating the PFO tunnel (c and d arrows). Usually, dual umbrella devices are used for PFO closure (e and f arrows), which compress and partially fill the PFO tunnel and stabilise interatrial septum.

Ao: aorta; IVC: inferior vena cava; SVC: superior vena cava.

Table 3. Overview of the epidemiology, diagnosis and management of acute PE associated with right heart thrombus or PFO.

Acute PE and right heart thrombus	Acute PE and PFO
How common is it?	
Right heart thrombi are detected in around 4% of unselected patients with acute PE and in up to 17% of patients with high-risk PE.	PFO is present in around 25% of adults in the general population and in a similar proportion of patients presenting with acute PE.
When should I suspect it?	
High-risk PE, i.e., PE presenting with cardiac arrest, obstructive shock, or persistent hypotension, carries an increased risk of right heart thrombus.	Symptoms and/or signs of a paradoxical embolism, most notably focal neurological deficit from a TIA or stroke.
An incidental finding of a filling defect in the right heart chambers on CTPA should be followed up immediately with confirmatory imaging, e.g., contrast echocardiography.	Hypoxaemia refractory to oxygen supplementation due to the right-to-left shunt.
	Clinical complications related to PFO in acute PE are more common in the presence of right ventricular dysfunction.
How is the diagnosis confirmed?	
Transthoracic echocardiography with or without microsphere contrast. Transoesophageal echocardiography is an alternative in ventilated patients, e.g., on the intensive care unit.	A "bubble" study by transthoracic echocardiography, using an agitated solution and Valsalva manoeuvre.
Contrast enhanced CMR may have superior sensitivity and specificity and allows differentiation from other intra-cardiac masses but should be reserved for stable patients.	Transoesophageal echocardiography is the gold-standard test and has better sensitivity and specificity than transthoracic imaging.
How does it change the management of PE?	
Current guidelines for the diagnosis and management of acute PE do not account for the presence of right heart thrombus when providing recommendations regarding reperfusion therapy.	Management of acute PE is similar with and without a co-existing PFO.
Right heart thrombus in the setting of acute PE may be an indicator of an adverse prognosis. There is a risk of further embolisation of material from the right heart chambers to the lung, especially with type A thrombus. Some experts will therefore treat these patients more aggressively.	In cases requiring percutaneous catheter-directed treatment, there is a theoretical risk of catheter-derived thrombus causing a paradoxical embolism.
The role of reperfusion therapy, including thrombolysis and catheter-directed therapy, prolonged anticoagulation, thrombophilia screening and vena cava filters in patients with acute PE and right heart thrombus remains unclear.	PFO closure is indicated when acute PE is complicated by paradoxical embolism in the presence of a PFO.

Notes: CMR: cardiac myocardial resonance imaging; CTPA: computed tomography pulmonary angiography; PE: pulmonary embolism; PFO: patent foramen ovale; TIA: transient ischaemic attack.

Percutaneous closure of a PFO is indicated when acute PE is complicated by paradoxical embolism (Figure 2), and surgical ligation may be considered if surgical embolectomy is performed, especially when combined with extra-corporeal membrane oxygenation, although the benefit of closure in reducing right-to-left shunting, refractory hypoxaemia and the risk of paradoxical embolism needs to be set against the benefit of the PFO acting as a pressure relief or "pop-off" valve in the context of right ventricular failure. Closure of a PFO in patients with Eisenmenger-like physiology (severe pulmonary hypertension and net right-to-left shunting) may precipitate acute RV failure and haemodynamic decompensation.

Prognostic Implications of PFO in PE

The presence of right-to-left shunting through a PFO has been associated with increased mortality in the setting of an acute PE. In one prospective study examining acute "major" PE, defined as PE with evidence of acute right ventricular pressure overload or pulmonary hypertension on echocardiographic assessment or catheterisation, the presence of a PFO was associated with a two-fold increased risk of in-hospital mortality compared to patients without a PFO (Konstantinides *et al.*, 1998). The presence of a PFO was also associated with in-hospital morbidity, defined as the occurrence of ischaemic stroke, peripheral arterial embolism, major bleeding, or the need for intubation or cardiopulmonary resuscitation. PFO remained an independent predictor of mortality after correcting for baseline clinical characteristics and the presence of right-sided thrombi.

Table 3 provides a summary overview of concepts including epidemiology, diagnosis and management of acute PE associated with right heart thrombus or PFO.

Bibliography

Barrios, D. *et al.* (2016). Right heart thrombi in pulmonary embolism, *European Respiratory Journal*, 48(5), pp. 1377–1385. doi:10.1183/13993003.01044-2016.

Barrios, D. *et al.* (2017). Prognostic significance of right heart thrombi in patients with acute symptomatic pulmonary embolism: Systematic review and meta-analysis, *Chest*, 151(2), pp. 409–416. doi:10.1016/j.chest.2016.09.038.

Chockalingam, A. *et al.* (2021). Catheter-directed therapies for pulmonary embolism: Considerations for patients with patent foramen ovale, *Journal of*

Thrombosis and Thrombolysis, 51(2), pp. 516–521. doi:10.1007/s11239-020-02189-2.

European Working Group on Echocardiography and Kronik, G. (1989). The European Cooperative Study on the clinical significance of right heart thrombi, *European Heart Journal*, 10(12), pp. 1046–1059. doi:10.1093/oxfordjournals.eurheartj.a059427.

Konstantinides, S. *et al.* (1998). Patent foramen ovale is an important predictor of adverse outcome in patients with major pulmonary embolism, *Circulation*, 97(19), pp. 1946–1951. doi:10.1161/01.CIR.97.19.1946.

Konstantinides, S.V. *et al.* (2020). 2019 ESC guidelines for the diagnosis and management of acute pulmonary embolism developed in collaboration with the European Respiratory Society (ERS): The task force for the diagnosis and management of acute pulmonary embolism of the European Society of Cardiology (ESC), *European Heart Journal*, 41(4), pp. 543–603. doi:10.1093/eurheartj/ehz405.

Silvestry, F.E. *et al.* (2015). Guidelines for the echocardiographic assessment of atrial septal defect and patent foramen ovale: From the American Society of Echocardiography and Society for Cardiac Angiography and Interventions, *Journal of the American Society of Echocardiography*, 28(8), pp. 910–958. doi:10.1016/j.echo.2015.05.015.

https://doi.org/10.1142/9781800612778_0010

Chapter 10

Acute Pulmonary Embolism in Pregnancy

Elizabeth B. Gay

*Harvard Medical School, Division of Pulmonary Critical Care Medicine,
Brigham and Women's Hospital, Harvard Medical School,
Boston, MA, USA*

Abstract

Pulmonary emboli represent a common and potentially life-threatening
cause of dyspnoea in pregnancy. Despite improvements in our understanding of risk factors for PE and advances in management, they remain
a source of substantial maternal morbidity and mortality. In this chapter,
we will review the epidemiology, risk factors, diagnosis, risk stratification, and management of PE in pregnancy. We will highlight concerns
unique to pregnancy, including the broad differential for dyspnoea in
pregnancy and the choice of anticoagulants.

Case

A 27-year-old woman presents to the emergency room at 28 weeks of
gestation with the acute onset of dyspnoea and pleuritic chest pain. This
is her first pregnancy and it has been uncomplicated. Her past medical
history is notable for obesity and mild asthma, currently well controlled
on a beta-2 agonist taken only as needed. She notes the onset of dyspnoea

and pleurisy in the early morning hours and describes that the symptoms woke her from sleep. She has not noticed lower extremity oedema, fevers, cough, or palpitations. She has no recent sick contacts and is up to date on routine pregnancy care and vaccinations. She takes no medications and does not smoke or drink alcohol. There is no family history of venous thromboembolism (VTE).

On examination, she is alert and oriented, with a heart rate of 127 beats per minute and a blood pressure of 100/75 mm Hg. Her oxygen saturation by pulse oximetry is 92% on room air. Her lungs are clear to auscultation and her cardiac examination reveals a regular heart rhythm with a tachy-cardic rate. She has no lower extremity oedema or pain to extremity palpa-tion. Her gynaecologic examination is normal and foetal heart sounds are detected. Her physicians are concerned about a pulmonary embolism (PE) and are considering the next best steps in diagnosis and management.

Patients such as this one are the source of angst for many healthcare providers, who feel the burden of caring for two patients. In this chapter, we will review the epidemiology, diagnosis, and management of acute PE in pregnancy. We will consider the challenges in diagnosis in the setting of pregnancy and discuss management of both low and high-risk PE in this unique patient population.

Epidemiology

Pregnant women are 5–10 times more likely than non-pregnant women to experience VTE.

The pathogenesis of VTE in pregnancy includes a combination of all factors related to Virchow's triad. Venous stasis arises from a mechanical effect of the enlarging uterus and a decrease in venous return. Damage to vessel endothelium may occur both during uncomplicated delivery and in the setting of hypertension related to pre-eclampsia or eclampsia. Finally, the thrombophilia of pregnancy is complex and involves increased fibrin production, decreased fibrinolysis, increased levels of factor II, VII, VIII, and X, and a decrease in anti-coagulant protein S levels. There is also acquired resistance to activated protein C.

The thrombophilia of pregnancy is evolutionarily adaptive as mater-nal haemorrhage remains the leading cause of maternal mortality world-wide. In the United States, acute PE is the leading cause of maternal mortality, with a mortality rate of 16 per 100,000 live births. The highest risk of death is up to 12 weeks post-partum, with 1/3–2/3rds of cases of VTE occurring after delivery. In recent years, the incidence of DVTs in pregnancy has declined, but deaths from PE remain unchanged.

In terms of preventing the devastating event of maternal death from PE, an understanding of which patients are at highest risk can aid in recognition and prevention. Established risk factors for VTE in pregnancy include multiple births, obesity, maternal age greater than 35, eclampsia or pre-eclampsia, Caesarean-section, haemorrhage, prior superficial venous thrombosis, smoking, hypertension, and heritable thrombophilia. Heritable thrombophilia is a relatively rare cause and most PEs in pregnancy happen in patients without a history of prior VTE. In terms of modifiable risk factors, smoking is likely the most important and all pregnant women should receive counselling and support for smoking cessation. Smoking cessation can also have a beneficial effect on other maternal and foetal health outcomes. Large database studies suggest that death from PE is more common in black patients of all ages. This disparity may reflect comorbidities, confounding factors, or additional genetic factors not yet well understood.

Universal prophylaxis for VTE in pregnancy is not recommended because of concern for bleeding complications. Pharmacologic prophylaxis is recommended if there is a prior history of VTE or known thrombophilia. Based on concerns detailed below about foetal safety and peripartum issues, the general recommendation for prophylaxis involves the use of low molecular weight heparin (LMWH). Guidelines suggest a duration of prophylaxis extending at least 6 weeks post-partum with consideration of 3 months post-partum for high-risk patients. Table 1 provides examples of known risk factors for PE in pregnancy.

Diagnosis

Symptoms, ECG, and laboratory testing

VTE is common and important to diagnose in pregnancy, but diagnosis can be challenging in part because symptoms are often non-specific. Dyspnoea is very common in normal pregnancies. Increases in progesterone and oestrogen increase minute ventilation, which may cause a sense of dyspnoea in the absence of pathology. Additional pathological causes of dyspnoea include asthma, anaemia, and heart failure. Relatively

Table 1.   Risk factors for PE in pregnancy.

Risk factor	
Personal history of VTE	• History of VTE related to pregnancy or oestrogen use • Transient risk factor induced PE or proximal DVT • Spontaneous distal calf DVT • Transient risk factor induced distal calf DVT • Recurrent VTE or recent VTE (<2 years)
Thrombophilia	• Known thrombophilia • Anti-phospholipid antibody syndrome • No thrombophilia detected but family history of severe VTE
Other risk factors	• Bed rest • Twin pregnancy • Post-partum infection • Age >35 • BMI >30 • Smoking

few pregnant patients with PE have oxygen saturations lower than 90%, so a normal oxygen saturation does not rule out PE in this situation. As opposed to their role in non-pregnant patients, clinical decision rules do not have a primary role in diagnosing PE in pregnancy as they seem to be less effective in helping clinicians decide who needs additional testing.

D-dimer is a laboratory measure of the degradation product of fibrin and has a role in excluding VTE in most low-risk outpatients. However, there are no established normal values for D-dimer in pregnancy and D-dimer may be elevated even in an uncomplicated pregnancy. Because pregnant patients were excluded from studies using D-dimer to rule out PE, it should not be used alone to rule out PE in pregnancy. As discussed in the following, it may have a role in more comprehensive decision frameworks. Additional studies of biomarkers for diagnosis of PE in pregnancy have been disappointing.

An ECG should be obtained to look for ischaemia or arrhythmia but will often show non-specific changes. The most common finding in PE is sinus tachycardia, but findings of RV strain may occur in higher-risk PE and should prompt further risk stratification, as described in the following.

The differential diagnosis of PE in pregnancy includes normal physiologic changes of advancing pregnancy, worsening of underlying lung disease (asthma, pulmonary hypertension), or cardiomyopathy. A physical exam may provide evidence of an alternative diagnoses and a clear explanation for dyspnoea may obviate the need to rule out PE. However, in most cases, physical exam, ECG, and laboratory work alone will not rule in another diagnosis and imaging will be required.

Imaging

Because symptoms, physical examination, and laboratory values are rarely adequate for the diagnosis of PE in pregnancy, the clinician will typically need to decide on additional testing. Treatment should be started while awaiting results of testing if there is a high clinical suspicion for PE.

In the presence of signs or symptoms of DVT, a compression ultrasound study with doppler flow analysis has a high yield for diagnosis and may obviate further testing. Because a delay in diagnosis increases the risks of poor outcomes, if ultrasound is not available quickly it is reasonable to proceed with a ventilation–perfusion (V/Q) scan or computed tomographic pulmonary angiography (CTPA).

Although a chest X-ray to start is reasonable to evaluate for alternative diagnoses and to allow interpretation of a V/Q scan, it cannot alone be used to rule in PE. The choice of additional imaging depends upon availability and institutional experience as both V/Q scans and CTPAs are reasonable studies. A V/Q scan is a nuclear test which uses a perfusion scan to show blood flow distribution and a ventilation scan to show airflow distribution in the lungs. One segmental or two subsegmental perfusion defects with a normally ventilated area (V/Q mismatch) is the definition of a high-probability scan for PE. V/Q scans are often diagnostic in pregnancy (up to 80% of the time) and minimise radiation. V/Q has the best diagnostic accuracy when the accompanying chest X-ray is normal, which is expected to be the case for most young pregnant patients. Estimates of the rate of diagnostic V/Q scans (either normal, low probability, or high probability scans) in pregnant patients range about 75–95%.

CTPA may be more readily available than V/Q scans in many institutions. The increased blood volume and cardiac output in pregnancy make quantifying and timing the intravenous contrast bolus more difficult, but a properly timed study has a high diagnostic yield and excellent negative predictive value. Studies estimating the rate of diagnostic CTPAs in pregnant patients range widely, with an average of about 80%. CTPA is preferred over a V/Q scan if a chest X-ray is abnormal. The radiation doses required by CTPA have not been found to present an increased risk of foetal death or developmental abnormalities and it remains an appropriate test for evaluating PE in pregnancy.

Several clinical diagnostic algorithms incorporating imaging have been evaluated in pregnant patients. The YEARS algorithm performed well in this population and includes ordering a D-dimer and then stratifying patients by whether they have any of the following: haemoptysis, clinical signs of DVT, or clinical suspicion of PE as the most likely diagnosis. CTPA is then performed based on a combination of D-dimer results and number of criteria met. Using this risk stratification, CTPA can be avoided in a substantial number of patients who will not go on to develop clinically relevant VTE (Figure 1).

Risk stratification

The consequences of PE range from trivial to life-threatening. Mortality is typically caused by extensive obstruction and subsequent haemodynamically instability, defined as shock. The mortality of so-called massive of high-risk PE approaches 50% in some series and up to 7% of PEs in pregnancy may present in this fashion.

Risk stratification for all patients with PE is based on the concept that the major cause of death in PE is from right ventricular (RV) strain and failure. Hence, risk stratification tools evaluate the impact of clot on the RV. The definition of massive PE includes the following: cardiac arrest, or obstructive shock as manifested by shock (end-organ damage, or persistent hypotension (SBP <90 or a drop from baseline of at least 40)) without another cause. It is important to rule out other causes of shock (sepsis, bleeding, atrial fibrillation) before assuming PE is responsible for haemodynamic decompensation. In pregnancy, end organ damage includes signs of foetal distress and this may be the earliest sign of decompensation.

Intermediate risk or sub-massive PE refers to patients who are haemodynamically stable but who have laboratory, echocardiographic, or imaging evidence of RV strain. This may manifest as abnormally elevated

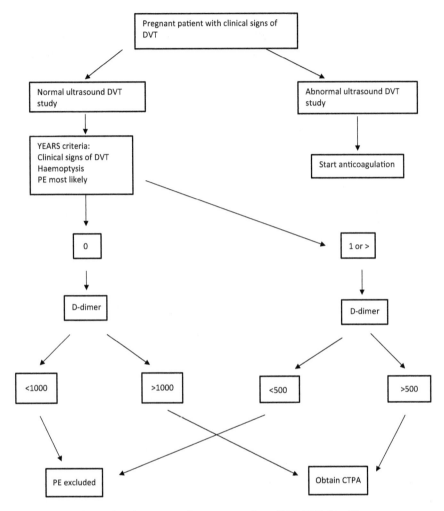

Figure 1.   Summary of pregnancy adapted YEARS algorithm.

laboratory values, specifically troponin T or I, BNP or N-terminal pro-BNP. These laboratory parameters should not be substantially different at baseline in pregnant populations and can still be used for risk stratification. Echocardiographic evidence of RV strain includes RV dilation, increased RV:LV ratio, increased RV systolic pressure (estimated from the tricuspid regurgitation jet), and decreased tricuspid annular plane of systolic excursion (TAPSE). A decrease in TAPSE suggests a decrease in RV function. A regional decline in RV function with free wall hypokinesis and apical sparing (the McConnell sign) is a specific finding for acute RV strain (though not specific for acute PE). A ratio of RV to LV end diastolic diameter of greater than 0.9 predicts an increased risk of a poor outcome. Additional findings of RV strain may be evaluated on more in-depth echocardiographic evaluation and include measurements of right ventricular fractional area of change, another marker of RV function. CT imaging findings suggesting right heart strain include RA enlargement, RV enlargement with septal bowing into the LV, and a ratio of RV to LV size of greater than 0.9. Patients with submassive (intermediate-risk) PE have a higher risk of decompensation and merit inpatient care with telemetry monitoring. For pregnant patients, foetal monitoring should be provided, if available.

Treatment

When there is a high clinical suspicion for acute PE, empiric anticoagulant therapy is indicated prior to the diagnostic evaluation, assuming no absolute contraindications exist.

Heparin products, which do not cross the placenta, remain the mainstay of anticoagulation in pregnancy. LMWHs have the advantage of a reliable and quick time to achieving anticoagulation and are recommended except where patients are close to delivery, or where concern exists around bleeding, severe renal insufficiency, or anticipated need for an invasive procedure. Higher doses of heparins are generally needed in pregnancy given alterations in plasma volume, GFR, and metabolism. Warfarin is generally avoided given known teratogenicity early in pregnancy and a higher risk of bleeding complications close to term. There is little data about the safety of novel oral anticoagulants in pregnancy and they should generally be avoided.

Anticoagulation is typically held in anticipation of delivery, with timing depending on the indication. Of note, neuraxial anaesthesia cannot be offered on full anticoagulation so the anticoagulation plan should be discussed in advance with the entire medical team. After delivery, anticoagulation can typically be resumed within 12 hours. For patients in whom there is a concern over the interruption of anticoagulation, assessment for lower extremity clot and consideration of a temporary IVC filter is reasonable. Duration of anticoagulation for the therapy of PE in pregnancy should be at least 3 months, with at least 6 weeks of post-partum antico-agulation. For patients with additional VTE risk factors beyond preg-nancy, duration should be individualised and may need to be longer.

Acutely, heparin therapy alone is appropriate for the majority of patients with low risk and intermediate risk PE in pregnancy. There is a general lack of data for the use of catheter-directed thrombolysis or mechanical clot extraction devices in pregnancy, and these interventions cannot be routinely recommended. There may be special circumstances in which these interventions are indicated for massive PE cases in which systemic thrombolysis is specifically contra-indicted. For patients with massive PE, observational data suggest that systemic thrombolysis and surgical thrombectomy are reasonable approaches, with acceptable risk of bleeding and foetal loss. Although concerns about lytic therapy in preg-nancy include effects on the maternal circulation (haemorrhage) and the placenta (abruption, fetal loss), thrombolytics do not cross the placenta in large amounts and this aggressive therapy may be life-saving in the setting of massive PE. Clinicians should prepare for substantial bleeding prior to delivery in the setting of thrombolysis and a multidisciplinary team approach will benefit patients.

Rescue therapy

There is little data to guide rescue therapy for pregnant patients with refractory shock despite attempts at thrombolysis. Case series describe patients rescued with VA-ECMO in the setting of cardiac arrest and for massive PE as a bridge to reperfusion using thrombolysis or surgical thrombectomy. These series not only describe high rates of bleeding (in around 50% of patients) but also reasonable maternal (70–80%) and foetal survival (60–70%). In general, when considering the pregnant patient with a massive PE, early involvement of multiple specialties including obstet-rics, thoracic surgery, cardiology, or interventional radiology, and poten-tially an ECMO team is recommended so that all options can be explored.

Outcomes and Case Follow-Up

Although thrombophilia appears to be a risk factor for early foetal loss, the maternal and foetal outcomes of appropriately diagnosed and treated PE in pregnancy are reasonably good.

Overall, the data suggest that both appropriate prevention for high-risk patients and early diagnosis and treatment will improve maternal mortality from VTE.

The young woman in our case had laboratory values which were unremarkable except for a mildly elevated BNP. She was started on a heparin infusion based on high clinical suspicion for VTE, and then underwent V/Q scintigraphy which was interpreted as high probability. Echocardiogram showed mild RV dilation, but no significant RV dysfunction. She was admitted for foetal monitoring for a few days, then discharged on enoxaparin. After delivery of a healthy boy at term, she completed 3 additional months of anticoagulation.

Summary

Pregnancy is an established risk factor for VTE, and acute PE is an important cause of maternal mortality. A high index of suspicion is required to diagnose PE in pregnancy because symptoms may overlap with symptoms of normal pregnancy. When there is a high clinical suspicion for PE, therapy with heparin should be initiated while awaiting confirmatory testing, which may include a V/Q scan or CTPA. As in non-pregnant patients, risk stratification for PE includes evaluation for signs of RV strain. For the rare but life-threatening case of massive PE in pregnancy, a multidisciplinary approach to discuss the risks and benefits of options for clot removal is recommended.

Bibliography

American Society of Hematology (ASH) (2018). Guidelines for management of venous thromboembolism — Venous thromboembolism in the context of pregnancy. American Society of Hematology 2018 guidelines for management of venous thromboembolism: Prophylaxis for hospitalized and non-hospitalized medical patients, *Blood Advances*, 2, pp. 3198–3225.

Blondon, M. *et al.* (2021). Management of high-risk pulmonary embolism in pregnancy, *Thrombosis Research*, 204, pp. P57–P65.

Dargaud, Y., Rugeri, L., Fleury, C. *et al.* (2017). Personalized thromboprophylaxis using a risk score for the management of pregnancies with high risk of thrombosis: A prospective clinical study, *Journal of Thrombosis Haemostasis*, 15, pp. 897–906.

Marik, P.E. and Plante, L.A. (2008). Venous thromboembolic disease in pregnancy, *New England Journal of Medicine*, pp. 359, 2025.

Van Der, P., Liselotte, M. *et al.* (2019). Pregnancy-adapted YEARS algorithm for diagnosis of suspected pulmonary embolism, *New England Journal of Medicine*, 380(12), pp. 1139–1149.

Chapter 11

Recurrent PE on Anticoagulation — What Should I Do Differently?

Karen A. Breen and Bhashkar Mukherjee

Guy's and St Thomas' NHS Foundation Trust, London, UK

Abstract

Patients with recurrent pulmonary embolism present unique challenges in management with ascertainment of anticoagulation compliance key to the determination of appropriate treatment. The use of risk stratification tools may be acceptable however this carries with it recognised limitations with a lack of validation for commonly used pre-test probability assessment tools. This chapter reviews recommended diagnostic strategies in patients with suspected recurrent pulmonary embolism focussing on appropriate imaging techniques, thrombophilia and cancer screening, advice around assessment of anticoagulation compliance, switching anticoagulation strategies, and prioritising those for follow up with appropriate assessment of risk of recurrence. Consideration around down-titration of dose for long-term anticoagulation is also included in patients with higher risk for bleeding.

Introduction

Recurrent PE on anticoagulant therapy is uncommon and occurs in up to 2% of patients on anticoagulation. The majority of patients presenting with acute recurrent PE will likely receive adjustment to their current treatment, often with escalation of their current anticoagulation to prevent thrombus extension and embolisation in order to reduce morbidity and mortality. Mechanical methods such as thrombectomy and/or local thrombolysis to remove thrombus may also be considered depending on the severity of the presentation. Few studies address management of anticoagulation in patients with recurrent venous events, specifically PE. Immediate management including anticoagulant choice will be influenced mainly by the circumstances leading to the recurrence and particularly whether the event occurred despite anticoagulation.

Investigations

The approach to diagnosing an episode of recurrent PE is similar to that used in the diagnosis of a first PE with the additional considerations of adequacy of the preceding anticoagulation and perhaps greater attention to the possible presence of chronic thrombotic disease and related complications. In diagnosing the recurrent event, historical considerations provide valuable early direction for management.

Diagnosis of Acute (Recurrent) PE

Taking a thorough history is crucial to try to determine a possible cause for recurrence, particularly determining if the event has occurred despite appropriate anticoagulation, i.e., treatment failure. It is important to ensure it is not labelled as a treatment failure if the recurrence is due to non-adherence to medication. Firstly, confirmation that the presentation is truly a recurrent event is important — comparison with previous imaging and consideration of symptoms should determine if this is a definite new VTE presentation. Additionally, whether already taking anticoagulation or not, a recurrent thrombosis will necessitate consideration of the possibility of chronic thromboembolic disease, which will have bearing on the presenting history, interpretation of investigations, and management for the individual.

The history should try to establish any chronicity of symptoms more than 2 weeks prior to the acute presenting event, the degree of recovery of symptoms after the previous PE along with duration and adherence to anticoagulation. There are data to suggest that with recurrence is slightly

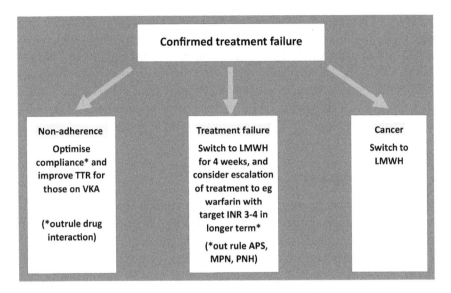

Figure 1.   Potential outcomes following confirmation of acute PE treatment failure.

more common with PE compared to deep vein thrombosis when the initial event was also a PE.

Commonly, the patient will be familiar with the symptom profile of PE and the history should aim to distinguish if there are chronic stable symptoms from or even prior to the initial PE event. There may be slow or only partial recovery after the initial PE meaning clarification around the presence of identifiable new symptoms with relation to anticoagulant use is important. The aim is to effectively distinguish between non-adherence and treatment failure and therefore, if this presentation represents a new acute PE after full recovery, acute on chronic PE, stable chronic thromboembolic disease, CTEPH, or another condition mimicking PE presentation (Figure 1).

Use of Clinical Pre-Test Probability Assessment Tools

Clinical decision rules to assess the pre-test probability of acute PE were not specifically designed with recurrent PE in mind but rather consider the clinical probability of the thrombotic event itself. The commonly used Wells rule, PERC (PE Rule out Criteria), and the Geneva score all include a history of previous VTE as part of their algorithm and give this factor a high weighting to reflect the higher implicit risk when there is such a history. The Caprini Model offers such a role in surgical patients to estimate risk of VTE. The YEARS score which is a simplified derivation from the Wells rule, does not include a history of PE but rather the clinician's overall impression of likelihood of PE and can help to exclude VTE without the need for imaging.

Use of Biomarkers

There is increasing interest in the use of biomarkers to provide an individualised assessment of risk of VTE, and they continue to have a place in the immediate assessment of a new recurrent event. D-dimer is commonly used and is part of standard guidelines for assessing an acute PE thanks to its high negative predictive value. It may be however elevated in many other conditions (including infection, pregnancy, malignancy, and cardiovascular disease) which complicates its interpretation in the acute setting. Nevertheless, it is included in most clinical prediction tools and more recently variable D-dimer cut-offs have been incorporated into tools such as the YEARS score.

D-dimer measured after a period of anticoagulation has also been used to predict risk of recurrence after a first unprovoked VTE event but this approach is not used routinely to the confounding factors in its interpretation. Despite negative post-treatment D-dimer levels, some 5% of the patients go on to have VTE recurrence. Where a negative D-dimer does not appear to change the risk profile significantly, seen especially in males, its use to exclude VTE recurrence is not recommended. It is also worth noting the lack of standardisation of commercially available D-dimer tests can lead to misclassification of risk.

Factor VIII has recently been associated with unprovoked as well as provoked VTE recurrence but its measurement should not be employed in isolation for predicting recurrent VTE. C-reactive protein (CRP) is routinely used as a marker of inflammation in the acute setting and is increasingly recognised for its role in thrombo-inflammation, particularly in monomeric form (mCRP) in the context of arterial thrombosis and myocardial reperfusion. There is evidence that native CRP as a biomarker of acute arterial thrombosis may carry association with venous thrombosis. Given its widespread use in acutely unwell patients and problems around non-specific interpretation, CRP measurement does not have a place in routine assessment of acute PE or risk of recurrence.

Imaging in Acute (Recurrent) PE

Imaging undertaken to assess for recurrent PE is directed at diagnosing and intervening on the new acute PE event, establishing the presence of and planning management of residual or chronic thrombotic disease or, with its exclusion, planning management in the absence of residual thrombotic disease.

In the acute setting, there is no validated standard as to which imaging modality to use for diagnosing or excluding acute recurrent PE. However, there are data to support use of both V/Q and CTPA imaging. Since the question is often whether the previous thrombotic load has resolved or if there is new or further thrombus it may be reasonable to repeat the imaging modality used for the first event to allow easier comparison between investigations.

If there is no historical imaging available, where there is low clinical likelihood of a chronic or recurrent acute PE, and especially in the absence of pre-existing lung parenchymal disease, V/Q SPECT is helpful as it has high negative predictive value to allow exclusion of thrombotic disease. Conversely, CT imaging allows consideration of other diagnoses where acute PE may not be all that likely. In practice, the choice of modality may be affected by both patient factors and local availability of imaging.

In the investigation and management of chronic thromboembolic pulmonary hypertension (CTEPH), both V/Q SPECT and CTPA have a role. V/Q-SPECT is advocated in current guidelines as the image modality of choice for excluding CTEPH; however, CTPA has the additional advantage of identifying features of both acute and chronic thrombotic disease. It also allows identification of CT features of right ventricular strain and tends to be more readily available in the setting of acute PE recurrence.

CT features indicating chronic thrombotic disease include eccentric or calcified thrombus, pulmonary arterial bands and webs, partial recanalisation of thrombus, and post-stenotic dilatation. There may also be systemic collateralisation from the bronchial circulation with prominent bronchial artery hypertrophy. Features suggestive of pulmonary hypertension include enlargement of the pulmonary arteries, narrowing or "pruning" of peripheral pulmonary arteries, pulmonary arterial calcification, tortuous pulmonary vessels and right ventricular enlargement, and hypertrophy. Additionally, there may be mosaic perfusion of the parenchyma reflecting heterogeneity of parenchymal blood flow.

Where available, echocardiography may play an important role in diagnosis. As described elsewhere, features of right ventricular strain and pulmonary hypertension are sought in this situation. With recurrent PE, there may already be right ventricular remodelling following the index presentation or evidence for ongoing persistent thromboembolic disease.

Why was There a Recurrence?

Non-compliance

Patients presenting with PE recurrence may be taking any form of anticoagulation including direct oral anticoagulants (DOACs), low molecular weight heparin (LMWH), vitamin K antagonist (VKA), e.g., warfarin or less commonly used agents such as fondaparinux.

Adherence tools may be useful to determine if the patient is simply not taking their medication as prescribed, and to encourage them to take their medications going forward. Checking dispensing records and questioning the patient may be helpful to determine non-adherence. Real world data have suggested adherence rates of <50% in patients taking DOACs for atrial fibrillation.

For those patients taking warfarin or a VKA, establishing the recent time in therapeutic range (TTR) is important, and whether, in the lead up to the diagnosis, the INR was subtherapeutic. Most patients on a VKA will have a target INR range between 2 and 3, and expected TTR of at least 60–70%. It is accepted it can be often difficult to achieve an expected TTR given the potential for food and drug interactions with warfarin/VKA. For those patients established on DOACs, there are many dosing recommendations depending on the agent used, as discussed in the following.

Screening for thrombophilia

Many patients presenting with a recurrent PE will already have investigations performed following the original event. Screening for an underlying thrombophilia associated with increased risk of recurrence is crucial.

Table 1. Antiphospholipid syndrome: Diagnostic criteria.

- Presence of lupus anticoagulant (LA)
- IgG or IgM anticardiolipin antibodies (aCL) present in medium or high titre (i.e., >40 GPL or MPL or >99th percentile)
- Anti-$\beta_2$glycoprotein-1 (aβ_2GPI) (IgG and/or IgM) >99th percentile

These aPL antibodies should be persistent, defined as being present on two or more consecutive occasions at least 12 weeks apart.

Antiphospholipid syndrome (APS) is particularly relevant given its particular association with recurrent VTE (Table 1). It is also important to exclude for those patients presenting with recurrent PE while taking a DOAC. Many of the inherited thrombophilia such as factor V Leiden heterozygosity or prothrombin gene mutation heterozygosity do not predict an increased risk of recurrence. Excluding less common prothrombotic conditions such as myeloproliferative disorders or paroxysmal nocturnal haemoglobinuria (PNH) are also important in this setting, since they may be a cause for recurrent thrombosis and warrant appropriate management with medications other than anticoagulation. Heparin-induced thrombocytopenia (HIT) is also worth considering in those patients taking LMWH.

Screening for cancer

Screening for malignancy should be considered in the absence of an alternative explanation. Patients will more than likely already have had thoracic imaging to confirm the diagnosis of PE, so abdominal and pelvic imaging should be completed where appropriate. Women should complete mammography if not performed recently and a PSA should be measured in males.

Management of the Acute (Recurrent) PE

The key decisions will relate to the acute management of recurrent PE, the subsequent choice and duration of anticoagulation and of course the additional longer-term strategies available for treatment of chronic thrombotic disease with and without pulmonary hypertension.

How is Anticoagulation Managed in Patients with Recurrent PE in the Acute Setting?

In the acute setting, when a new PE recurrence is confirmed in the context of adequate prior anticoagulation, usually patients will be managed with a switch to therapeutic dose LMWH while investigations around the underlying cause are carried out. Following the acute presentation, for patients in whom recurrence occurred despite treatment with a DOAC, a switch to warfarin is often considered (discussed later).

In the setting of acute VTE, an initial loading dose of Rivaroxaban 15 mg twice daily is recommended for the first three weeks, with 20 mg once daily advised thereafter for the first 6 months. This is followed by a dose decreased to 10 mg once daily in those patients felt not to be at high risk of recurrence. Similarly, Apixaban is recommended at a loading dose of 10 mg twice daily in the first week, followed by a dose of 5 mg twice daily in the first 6 months, with a decreased dose recommended in anyone needing long-term anticoagulation of 2.5 mg twice daily. Finally, the recommended dose of Edoxaban is 60 mg once daily. There are further dose changes recommended in patients with renal impairment, while extremes of body weight may also have a bearing. A secondary prevention dose of dabigatran 150 mg twice daily is recommended.

Administration of most medications is not dependent on co-administration with food except for Rivaroxaban. Patient registries have shown there is often variation in dosing prescribed to patients because of perceived bleeding risk and in some cases, patients may not be receiving the appropriate dose recommendation.

Checking for potential drug interactions is also required since some concomitant medications may lead to a decreased anticoagulant effect.

For those patients, in whom there is a concern about significant progression despite optimal anticoagulation in the acute setting, an inferior vena cava (IVC) filter may need to be considered. However, in practice their use remains limited and are often not advisable given the possibility of device thrombosis or migration.

Follow-Up and Long-Term Management

Risk of recurrence

At the presentation of their index thrombotic event, most patients should have had some assessment of the possible risk factors for developing

VTE. In tandem, some consideration will usually have been given to their risk of recurrent thromboses as this will influence the type and duration of anticoagulation. In some cases, cessation of anticoagulation may be associated with an unacceptably high risk of VTE recurrence; this should trigger a discussion about eligibility for life-long anticoagulation taking into consideration the long-term individual bleeding risk of such a strategy.

Risk prediction models used to estimate the risk of recurrent PE provide a tool to aid decision-making in long-term anticoagulation management. In general terms, the risk of any VTE recurrence once anticoagulation has been stopped (after at least 3 months of treatment) is approximately 10% in the first year after treatment, 16% at 2 years, 25% at 5 years, and 36% at 10 years, with 4% of recurrent VTE events resulting in death. With extended anticoagulation, the risk reduces to around 7% cumulatively over 5 years. However, case fatality rates remaining significant at nearly 5% per year. This highlights the importance of both appropriate long-term anticoagulation and of recognition and management of recurrent cases.

Multiple transient and persistent risk factors as well as hereditary risk factors may all have a bearing on the specific risk of recurrent VTE for an individual. General prediction tools are available, such as the Vienna score, HERDOO2 score, and DASH scores, to quantitatively estimate relative risks of VTE recurrence. While they use different variables, rely on slightly different definitions of "unprovoked" VTE, and are reliant on specific D-dimer assays, these scoring systems are widely used. Men seem to be at higher risk of VTE recurrence if anticoagulation is stopped and the HERDOO2 score, for example, can help identify women in whom the risk is relatively lower. The Vienna prediction model identified a number of factors predisposing individuals to recurrence of VTE after a first unprovoked event in those without thrombophilic defects, creating a risk score to compare to a nomogram that assists in long-term anticoagulation decisions. The DASH score is a more simplified tool to calculate the risk of recurrent VTE in individuals who have completed a 3–6 month course of anticoagulation with a VKA. While these are useful tools to predict recurrence risk, they have only been validated in the setting of a first thrombotic event. They are therefore less useful in those who have already presented with a recurrence due to anticoagulation failure.

Post-anticoagulation imaging

In clinical practice, the use of compression ultrasound (CUS) to determine residual venous obstruction (RVO) post DVT is rationalised by the presence of persistent symptoms although there are some data to support its use as a routine clinical decision-making tool to refine an individual's risk of VTE recurrence.

Similar considerations can be invoked following a PE with the pro-active estimation of risk of PE recurrence in an individual through use of imaging after a period of anticoagulation. Following PE, the persistence of residual clot burden is known to reduce over time but this process is dependent upon a number of factors including the initial clot burden, the presence of chronic disease at initial diagnosis, and age (above 65 years). However, this has not been well studied in a systematic fashion, with a variety of imaging modalities and use of different assessment time-points during ongoing anticoagulation. Some 46–66% of patients have residual perfusion defects at 3 months and in up to 25% of patients, these persist at one year. This is important to appreciate given symptomatic improvement is also variable and tends to be often slower than may be appreciated, with 47% of patients also demonstrably deconditioned after a year in the only large cohort study to review this.

In practice, where anticoagulation has been well tolerated, most patients are currently recommended to continue indefinite anticoagulation treatment after "unprovoked" PE meaning the utility of re-imaging patients to refine anticoagulation management is not required.

Which long-term anticoagulation?

Choice of long-term anticoagulation will be based on the underlying cause for VTE recurrence. For those not related to adherence issues, and who were taking a DOAC, or VKA targeting an INR between 2 and 3 and TRR >60%, continuation of a VKA with an increased target INR of 3–4 is advised. Although not licensed, in practice, some clinicians may choose to use a higher dose of DOAC, e.g., apixaban 5 mg twice daily including if the recurrence occurred during a period of maintenance dose anticoagulation with Apixaban 2.5 mg twice daily. In the setting of cancer-associated thrombosis recurrence, titration of LMWH according to anti-Xa levels may be used. Close monitoring of these patients, especially in the initial phase is crucial to ensure the recurrence is adequately treated.

Conclusion

In patients presenting with potential recurrent PE, confirmation of a new thrombosis with imaging is imperative. Many recurrences are due to non-adherence to anticoagulation, but screening for malignancy needs careful consideration. Escalation of anticoagulation will only need consideration in a minority.

Bibliography

American Society of Hematology (ASH) (2018). Guidelines for management of venous thromboembolism — Venous thromboembolism in the context of pregnancy. American Society of Hematology 2018 guidelines for management of venous thromboembolism: Prophylaxis for hospitalized and nonhospitalized medical patients, *Blood Advances*, 2(3), pp. 198–225.

Antithrombotic therapy for VTE disease: Second update of the CHEST Guideline and Expert Panel Report. https://journal.chestnet.org/article/S0012-3692(21)01506-3/fulltext.

Chapter 12

Pulmonary Embolism with Contraindications to Anticoagulation — How to Proceed

Eileen Harder and Aaron B. Waxman

Division of Pulmonary Critical Care Medicine, Brigham and Women's Hospital, Harvard Medical School, Boston, MA, USA

Abstract

Acute pulmonary embolism (PE) can be associated with significant mortality, and the risk of death rises even further with delayed therapy. In selecting the optimal treatment, rapid assessment of disease severity is necessary; however, the risk of bleeding — the major complication of PE therapy — must also be carefully considered. In practice, bleeding risk spans a continuum, with the probability for a specific patient dependent on the required intervention itself, concurrent acute conditions, and certain prior comorbidities, among other factors. While the vast majority of patients with haemodynamically stable pulmonary emboli will be candidates for therapeutic anticoagulation, life-threatening disease may pose a complex challenge. In these situations, a structured approach to decision-making is necessary, with understanding of absolute contraindications to thrombolysis, anticipated benefits, and alternative treatment modalities. This chapter will discuss the management of patients with contraindications to systemic thrombolysis or to therapeutic anticoagulation, with particular focus on the populations with neurologic disease, pregnancy, and malignancy.

Introduction

Medical decision-making is a complex undertaking that ideally is rooted in high-quality research and comprehensive clinical evidence. In the absence of objective data, however, physicians are often forced to rely heavily on intuition and perhaps common sense. When the lack of evidence persists over time, it is not a surprise that these decisions evolve into standard practice. Regardless — and particularly when making vital management choices in the setting of a life-threatening condition such as a pulmonary embolism (PE) — it is important to understand the data underlying current guidelines and recommendations.

This chapter will review the contraindications to thrombolysis and anticoagulation in acute PE, with a focus on the existing literature in which these recommendations are based.

What is a Contraindication?

To begin, we need to understand the meaning of a contraindication to treatment. In simplest terms, contraindications are widely utilised constructs that simply and rapidly weigh the balance of risk versus benefit of a treatment or procedure to guide management decisions. Generally, two types are recognised: an absolute contraindication denotes the presence of severe and potentially life-threatening risks that prohibit use of an intervention under any circumstance; in contrast, a relative contraindication represents a condition that makes a treatment option possibly inadvisable.

Assessment of Bleeding Risk

The major risk of treatment in PE is bleeding. Following disease staging by risk stratification, all patients under consideration for any intervention — from anticoagulation to surgery to thrombolysis — should undergo a prompt assessment of bleeding risk. Certain conditions, such as pregnancy and cancer, warrant special consideration and are discussed later.

In the event of a contraindication to first-line therapy, a structured approach to management is critical. In these situations, the first question is whether that contraindication is relative or can be modified: hypertension can be controlled, for example, and while bleeding risk rises with age, this possibility may be considered acceptable in the face of severe haemodynamic instability. If the bleeding risk remains unacceptably high, however, the focus should shift to availability and feasibility of alternate treatments, acknowledging that choices are generally limited.

In life-threatening VTE, systemic thrombolysis is widely accepted as the treatment of choice. When an absolute contraindication exists (Table 1), the choices are surgical embolectomy versus catheter-based approaches.

Surgical embolectomy is indicated in patients with haemodynamically unstable PE in whom thrombolytic therapy is prohibited, and it is generally recognised as the best option in those who fail thrombolysis. Catheter-directed therapies may also be an option in select patients. The choice between surgical and catheter-based approaches depends upon available expertise, patient-specific factors, and anticipated outcomes.

Table 1.   Contraindications to thrombolytic therapy.

Absolute Contraindications:
- Prior intracranial haemorrhage
- Known structural intracranial cerebrovascular disease
- Known malignant intracranial neoplasm
- Ischaemic stroke within last 3 months
- Suspected aortic dissection
- Active bleeding or bleeding diathesis
- Recent surgery encroaching on the spinal canal or brain
- Recent closed-head or facial trauma with radiographic evidence of bony fracture or brain injury

Relative Contraindications:
- Age >75 years
- PE in pregnancy
- Current use of anticoagulants
- Non-compressible vascular punctures
- Pericarditis or pericardial effusion
- Traumatic or prolonged CPR (>10 minutes)
- Recent internal bleeding (within 2–4 weeks)
- History of chronic, severe, and poorly controlled hypertension
- Severe uncontrolled hypertension *on presentation* (systolic >180 mmHg or diastolic >110 mmHg)
- Dementia
- Remote (>3 months) ischaemic stroke
- Major surgery within 3 weeks

In a small number of patients, even anticoagulation may pose an unacceptable risk. Retrievable inferior vena cava (IVC) filter insertion in acute PE can be considered if anticoagulation is contraindicated or if interruption is foreseen within a month of the acute PE. The use of retrievable filters is encouraged, and those should be removed within the recommended time interval, as late retrieval promotes complications including migration and thrombus propagation. While the exact timing is widely debated, it is generally accepted that filters should be extracted by 3–6 months post-placement. If possible, earlier retrieval should be considered if the contraindication to anticoagulation resolves beforehand.

In patients with acute PE who are able to receive anticoagulation, guidelines from the American College of Chest Physicians (ACCP) recommend against IVC filter insertion, although they acknowledge uncertainty regarding the risk and benefits in the subset with hypotension. There is no evidence to support routine placement of IVC filters in submassive PE and proximal deep venous thrombosis (DVT).

Management of VTE in the Neurologic or Neurosurgical Setting

In many cases, the risk of treatment is straightforward. When considering thrombolytic therapy, absolute neurologic contraindications to systemic and catheter-directed thrombolysis (CDT) centre upon cerebrovascular pathology, traumatic brain injury (TBI), and recent neurosurgery. Based on the use of thrombolytics in the setting of ischaemic stroke, transient ischaemic attack within 24 hours of presentation is also considered an absolute contraindication for thrombolysis, as even a relatively short period of ischaemia markedly increases vascular permeability and haemorrhagic transformation risk.

If a neurologic constraint precludes systemic thrombolysis in massive or high-risk PE, consideration should turn to surgical embolectomy or a catheter-based approach. In these situations, there are no data comparing safety and outcomes between these interventions, although surgical embolectomy provides a level of bleeding control that catheter-directed therapies do not. In cases where these approaches are being considered, management should depend on operator expertise and patient-specific risk factors. When reperfusion therapy is felt to be too dangerous, the subsequent decision on administration of anticoagulation relies on the ongoing neurologic pathology.

Among patients with ischaemic stroke, PE represents the most common cause of death in the weeks immediately following the acute event. Based on the European Society of Cardiology (ESC) and ACCP guidelines, a history of an ischaemic stroke within the past 3–6 months is an absolute contraindication to systemic thrombolysis. The risk of anticoagulation in this population, however, is not clearly defined, and even early low-dose heparin prophylaxis appears to increase the likelihood of haemorrhagic conversion. While anticoagulation initiation is generally delayed until two weeks post-ischaemic stroke for atrial fibrillation, there are conflicting recommendations regarding PE management: the National Health Service suggests it can be initiated in the acute period for proximal DVT or PE, while the American Heart Association (AHA) advises against it in moderate to severe stroke.

VTE is also a serious complication of traumatic and haemorrhagic brain disease. PE complicates the clinical course of up to 25% of patients who present with TBI, and treatment decisions must balance the inherent risks of thromboembolism against worsening intracranial haemorrhage. In those patients who will receive therapy, the initial timing and agent are important considerations. Most would recommend starting therapy as early as 48 hours from stable head imaging, allowing for establishment and maturation of intracranial clot to prevent uncontrolled bleeding. Given the extensive experience and easy reversibility, intravenous unfractionated heparin without an initial bolus is frequently the treatment of choice, with a therapeutic target partial thromboplastin time (PTT) of 60–80 seconds. Once the concern for bleeding has passed, patients can be transitioned to an oral agent. IVC filters can be considered in patients with proximal lower extremity DVT that are felt to be at exceptionally high risk for haemorrhagic complications or recurrent bleeding, have other systemic contraindications, or require surgical intervention.

Anticoagulation therapy for patients diagnosed with VTE in the early post-neurosurgical period causes significant angst due to the concern for ICH. While there is growing data on prophylaxis, in this population there is limited evidence to guide treatment of manifest VTE. In particular, there is little consensus to guide when it is safe to start anticoagulation post-operatively, although a wide range of intervals varying from 2 days to 30 days have been reported. Published studies are often based on relatively small numbers of patients; however, they suggest the timing of anticoagulation initiation does not significantly alter the rate of ICH after surgery in most cases.

Patients with metastatic or primary brain tumours represent a special situation: while they have a particularly high frequency of VTE, surgery in these cases also unfortunately imparts the greatest risk of intracranial bleeding with rates of 3–15%. Based on data from the American College of Surgeons National Surgical Quality Improvement Project, the estimated rate of DVT and PE was 2.4% and 1.3% in patients undergoing craniotomy, with 30-day mortality rates of 10.2% and 10.7%, respectively. Given the high risk of bleeding, systemic thrombolysis is not an option in this population, regardless of PE severity. There is growing evidence that patients with primary and metastatic brain tumours can be safely anticoagulated for VTE when carefully monitored. Of note, certain untreated tumours — particularly melanoma, thyroid, renal, and hepatocellular carcinomas — merit careful consideration and observation, as patients with these highly vascular lesions have higher rates of ICH compared to the general cancer population.

In treatment of VTE in the post-neurosurgical patient, most centres utilise unfractionated heparin as the first-line agent because it can be readily reversed in case of ICH. Therapy should be initiated 48 hours after surgery, with a therapeutic target range of 1.5–3 times the control activated PTT. Patients can be transitioned to an oral anticoagulant or maintained on low molecular weight heparin after a period of careful observation. Both rivaroxaban and apixaban showed similar efficacy and reduced rate of bleeding compared with warfarin and LMWH in cancer-related VTE. Of note, bleeding rates in patients treated with warfarin are significantly higher when compared to those who receive a direct oral anticoagulant. This is largely related to the underlying disadvantages of warfarin, including its vast potential for drug interactions and a narrow therapeutic range requiring frequent monitoring. Interestingly, the risk of bleeding complications with warfarin does not correlate with the target INR, warfarin dose, or time spent out of the therapeutic range.

Management of VTE in Pregnancy

Pregnancy is a well-described risk factor for VTE, with an approximate 4- to 5-fold increase in incidence compared to non-pregnant women. Estimates suggest that PE develops in 1–2 of 1,000 pregnancies. Notably, the immediate post-partum period also carries increased thrombotic risk: while more than half of VTE's occur during pregnancy, the rest take place largely in the 6 weeks following pregnancy. PE carries significant mortality implications during pregnancy, with a mortality rate of 1.1–1.5 per 100,000 women.

Pregnancy is considered a relative contraindication to thrombolysis because of the potential complications affecting both mother and foetus. Along with the same complications seen in non-pregnant women, there are additional obstetrical conditions to consider including uterine, placental, post-partum haemorrhage; spontaneous abortion of the foetus; and hematoma at the episiotomy site. Regardless, the existing literature does not suggest prohibitive risk associated with thrombolysis for PE in pregnancy; this therapy should be considered in massive or high-risk disease on a case-by-case basis. The approach to anticoagulation is addressed in a separate chapter.

Management of PE in the Setting of Cancer

Malignancy promotes hypercoagulability through cancer, treatment, and patient-specific mechanisms that ultimately culminate in an increased risk of VTE. Factors contributing to a prothrombotic state include abnormalities in coagulation, fibrinolysis and platelet function; blood flow stasis due to physical tumour compression of vessels; and aberrant endothelial injury or activation.

As noted earlier, intracranial cancers are considered an absolute contraindication to the use of thrombolytics. Anticoagulation, however, may be an option in this population, recognising that the risk of intracranial haemorrhage — even with metastatic disease to the brain — varies with cancer type and prior treatment.

Because of the apparent increased risk of bleeding, malignancies that do not involve the brain are considered a relative contraindication to thrombolysis. Notably, metastatic disease at the time of cancer diagnosis is one of the strongest predictors of VTE within the subsequent first year. Clinicians often withhold thrombolytics in patients with extracranial cancers and so the true incidence of bleeding with thrombolysis in patients with malignancy is not well studied. Most data are based on extensive retrospective data surveys of hospital system medical records; however, they confirm that patients with cancer are less likely to receive a thrombolytic and are more likely to die from VTE while in hospital.

CDT is an alternative approach for patients at increased risk of bleeding. CDT can allow for local but more focused thrombolytic injection, with reduced infusion times. In the general population, it is not clear as to the extent that CDT ameliorates bleeding risk and therefore whether it actually offers a safer approach than systemic thrombolysis. While evidence continues to grow, it is generally recognised that the risk of bleeding with CDT is still greater than that of anticoagulation alone, although likely less than thrombolysis. While the ACCP does recommend CDT for VTE, the recommendation is based on low-quality evidence, and they note that the balance of the risks and benefits with CDT is variable. Furthermore, this treatment has not been specifically evaluated in a population consisting exclusively of only cancer patients. Because of the concern for bleeding complications with either systemic or CDT, the use of these approaches should be considered on an individualised basis, with comparison of bleeding risk — incorporating tumour type, burden, location, among other patient specific factors — against that of death from VTE.

Conclusion

Morbidity and mortality remain high with VTE, particularly in the population where effective therapies may pose an unacceptably high risk of bleeding and death. Rapid risk stratification and bleeding risk assessment is critical for early management in acute PE. Notably, the spectrum of bleeding risk varies widely: at one extreme, there is the subset with exceptionally high risk comorbidities that are largely neurologic and preclude most treatment options, while the other end is occupied by patients who require extra consideration for some increased bleeding risk but who can receive most standard therapies. In these populations, decisions regarding early management — and in particular reperfusion treatment — should largely be made on a case-by-case basis with careful assessment of the potential risks and anticipated benefits.

Bibliography

Algattas, H., Kimmell, K.T., Vates, G.E., and Jahromi, B.S. (2015). Analysis of venous thromboembolism risk in patients undergoing craniotomy, *World Neurosurgery*, 84, pp. 1372–1379.

Condliffe, R., Elliot, C.A., Hughes, R.J., Hurdman, J., Maclean, R.M., Sabroe, I., van Veen, J.J., and Kiely, D.G. (2014). Management dilemmas in acute pulmonary embolism, *Thorax*, 69, pp. 174–180.

Cote, L.P., Greenberg, S., Caprini, J.A., Stone, J., Arcelus, J.I., Lopez-Jimenez, L., Rosa, V., Schellong, S., Monreal, M., and Investigators, R. (2014). Outcomes in neurosurgical patients who develop venous thromboembolism: A review of the RIETE registry, *Clinical and Applied Thrombosis Hemostasis*, 20, pp. 772–778.

de Melo Junior, J.O., Lodi Campos Melo, M.A., da Silva Lavradas, L.A.J., Ferreira Lopes, P.G., Luiz II, O., de Barros, P.L., da Mata Pereira, P.J., and Niemeyer Filho, P. (2020). Therapeutic anticoagulation for venous thromboembolism after recent brain surgery: Evaluating the risk of intracranial hemorrhage, *Clinical Neurology and Neurosurgery*, pp. 197, 106202.

Divito, A., Kerr, K., Wilkerson, C., Shepard, S., Choi, A., and Kitagawa, R.S. (2019). Use of anticoagulation agents after traumatic intracranial hemorrhage, *World Neurosurgery*, 123, pp. e25–e30.

Kabashneh, S., Alkassis, S., Shanah, L., and Alkofahi, A.A. (2020). Venous thromboembolism in patients with brain cancer: Focus on prophylaxis and management, *Cureus*, 12, pp. e8771.

Lin, R.J., Green, D.L., and Shah, G.L. (2018). Therapeutic anticoagulation in patients with primary brain tumors or secondary brain metastasis, *Oncologist*, 23, pp. 468–473.

Poupore, N., Strat, D., Mackey, T., Snell, A., and Nathaniel, T. (2020). Ischemic stroke with a preceding Trans ischemic attack (TIA) less than 24 hours and thrombolytic therapy, *BMC Neurology*, 20, pp. 197.

Prior, A., Fiaschi, P., Iaccarino, C., Stefini, R., Battaglini, D., Balestrino, A., Anania, P., Prior, E., and Zona, G. (2021). How do you manage ANTICOagulant therapy in neurosurgery? The ANTICO survey of the Italian Society of Neurosurgery (SINCH), *BMC Neurology*, 21, pp. 98.

Rodriguez, D., Jerjes-Sanchez, C., Fonseca, S., Garcia-Toto, R., Martinez-Alvarado, J., Panneflek, J., Ortiz-Ledesma, C., and Nevarez, F. (2020). Thrombolysis in massive and submassive pulmonary embolism during pregnancy and the puerperium: A systematic review, *The Journal of Thrombosis and Thrombolysis*, 50, pp. 929–941.

Scheller, C., Rachinger, J., Strauss, C., Alfieri, A., Prell, J., and Koman, G. (2014). Therapeutic anticoagulation after craniotomies: Is the risk for secondary hemorrhage overestimated? *Journal of Neurological Surgery Part A: Central European Neurosurgery*, 75, pp. 2–6.

Weeda, E.R., Hakamiun, K.M., Leschorn, H.X., and Tran, E. (2019). Comorbid cancer and use of thrombolysis in acute pulmonary embolism, *The Journal of Thrombosis and Thrombolysis,* 47, pp. 324–327.

Part 4

Follow-Up

Chapter 13

Anticoagulation: Which Agent and for How Long?

Charlie Lee and Karina C. Shuttie

Division of Pulmonary Critical Care Medicine, Brigham and Women's Hospital, Harvard Medical School, Boston, MA, USA

Abstract

This chapter provides insight into the clinical decision-making process when selecting an outpatient anticoagulation agent and length of therapy following acute pulmonary embolism, focusing on aspects such as patient risk factors, comorbidities, and socioeconomic barriers to guide clinical decisions, as well as reviewing the anticoagulation classes and their mechanisms to better understand choice of therapy. Additionally, this chapter discusses transient versus reversible causes of pulmonary embolism, as well as acquired versus heritable risk factors, which determine the length of anticoagulation therapy required.

Introduction

Once a pulmonary embolism (PE) has been identified and treated acutely, the work is not done. The patient must be sent home on an appropriate anticoagulation regimen with the right agent and planned duration of treatment. Risk of recurrence in a patient should guide clinical decision-making.

When it comes to choosing the right agent for a patient there are factors to consider beyond just efficacy; one must consider cost, compliance, access, and each patient's individual background and medical history. We encourage a holistic approach when assessing appropriate anticoagulation therapy with the goal of choosing a regimen a patient can realistically maintain. Each of the main categories of anticoagulants has their benefits and drawbacks, which we will explore further in this chapter.

Outpatient Anticoagulant Medication Classes

To date, there are four classes of anticoagulant to consider for outpatient PE management: vitamin K antagonists (VKAs), direct oral anticoagulants (DOACs) indirect thrombin inhibitors, and indirect factor Xa inhibitors (Figure 1). DOACs have two subclasses: direct factor Xa inhibitors and direct thrombin.

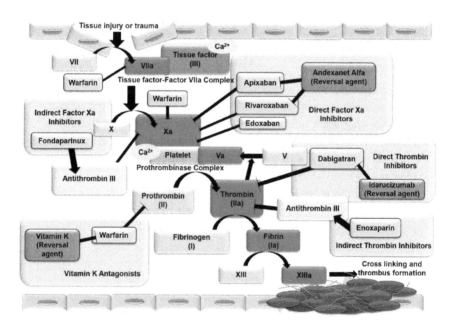

Figure 1. Extrinsic coagulation cascade and anticoagulant classes. There are four anticoagulation classes available for PE treatment and prevention: VKAs, DOACs, indirect thrombin inhibitors, and indirect factor Xa inhibitors. Direct factor Xa inhibitors and direct thrombin inhibitors are subclasses of DOACs.

Vitamin K antagonists

Traditionally, it was common practice to transition most patients from intravenous unfractionated heparin to oral VKAs as maintenance therapy for PE management. Warfarin is the most used VKA and works by competitively inhibiting the vitamin K epoxide reductase complex 1 (VKORC1). VKORC1 is primarily in the liver and helps activate vitamin K-dependent coagulation factors II (prothrombin), VII, IX, and X, through carboxylation. By blocking the function of VKORC1, these coagulation factors cannot function properly and are unable to bind calcium and phospholipid membranes needed to perform their clotting actions. It is important to note that this block of carboxylation occurs during protein synthesis and therefore does not affect the function of existing proteins. Thus, the anticoagulant effect of VKAs is delayed about 3 days, or about the time of the longest half-life of vitamin-K dependent factors, factor II, as you must wait for previously synthesised proteins to wash out. During this time, it is necessary to concurrently bridge the patient either with IV heparin or enoxaparin until their international normalised ratio (INR) is in therapeutic range for 2 consecutive days. Prothrombin time (PT) is not a reliable indication of therapeutic effect as PT will prolong first due to it being related to depletion of factor VII, which has a shorter half-life of 4–6 hours compared to 60 hours with factor II. In addition to its effect on clotting factors, VKAs also inhibit carboxylation of vitamin K dependent proteins c and s. These proteins selectively inhibit activated factors VIII and V; therefore, initiation of warfarin creates a transient procoagulant effect making heparin bridge even more critical.

What to consider when using VKAs?

Once a patient is discharged on warfarin, they will require close outpatient INR monitoring to ensure they remain within therapeutic range. This often requires a dedicated team of providers or an anticoagulation clinic to facilitate regular INR checks and adjust the warfarin dose accordingly. At first, your patient will require frequent INR checks until their INR is within therapeutic range for at least 2 consecutive weeks, then INR checks can be less frequently checked, i.e., every other week and eventually monthly.

Certain comorbidities can affect INR stability. As warfarin is mainly metabolised in the liver, hepatic disease may cause increased drug levels, decreased coagulation factors, and increased risk of bleeding. Warfarin is partly excreted through the kidneys and therefore dosing is often lowered in patients with renal disease; however, warfarin is the drug of choice in this population. Heart failure has also been found to interfere with INR stability which may increase bleeding risk. Acute illness can also alter effects of warfarin, especially infections or gastrointestinal illnesses. Warfarin also crosses the placenta with some reported teratogenic effects in first trimester exposures and it is contraindicated in pregnancy except for patients with mechanical valve replacements at high risk for thromboembolism.

It can be challenging to keep patients at a stable therapeutic INR range, as there are many potential dietary and drug effects that can interfere with the pharmacokinetics of warfarin. While on warfarin, patients will need to be educated on the effects of vitamin K has on their INR. It is important to counsel them on consuming a consistent level of vitamin K rich foods (Table 1) rather than eliminating them from their diet. Patients also need to keep in mind other additional vitamin K sources such as multivitamins and nutritional drinks. Due to the numerous drug-to-drug interactions with warfarin (Table 2), it is critical to counsel patients on the importance of reporting any new medication changes, especially antibiotics. Once you are aware of the medication change, it is important to check their INR while on treatment, then again after discontinuation and adjust the warfarin dose accordingly to maintain a therapeutic INR. Additionally, it is also important to counsel patients on avoiding excessive alcohol consumption and smoking while on warfarin.

Direct oral anticoagulants

In current practice, DOACs are the anticoagulants of choice due to their rapid onset and offset, no required monitoring, and fewer drug

Table 1. Examples of vitamin K rich foods. Vitamin K can reverse the effects of warfarin. Maintaining a consistent intake of vitamin K rich food is better than eliminating it from the diet.

Vitamin K rich foods		
High	**Medium**	**Low**
• Brussels sprout	• Asparagus	• Avocado
• Mustard greens	• Green beans	• Banana
• Collard greens	• Broccoli	• Corn
• Turnip greens	• Cabbage	• Fruit
• Spinach	• Carrots	• Potatoes
• Kale	• Cauliflower	• Tomatoes

Table 2. Examples of common VKA drug-to-drug interactions. Multiple antibiotics and various drug classes can increase or decrease the therapeutic effect of VKAs and affect bleeding and clotting risks.

Common VKA drug-to-drug interactions	
Increase therapeutic effect (↑ bleed risk)	**Decrease therapeutic effect (↑ clot risk)**
• Acetaminophen	• Vitamin K
• Xanthine oxidase inhibitors	• Antibiotics
• Androgens	o Dicloxacillin
• Antibiotics	o Nafcillin
o Cephalosporins	o Rifampin
o Fluoroquinolones	• Azathioprine
o Macrolides	• Carbamazepine
o Penicillins	• Cholestyramine
o Sulfa derivative	• Phenobarbital
• Azole antifungals	• St. John's Wort
• Cholesterol lowering agents	• Sucralfate
• Glucocorticosteroids	
• Proton pump inhibitors	
• Serotonin reuptake inhibitors	

interactions (Table 3). DOACs are categorised into two classes: direct factor Xa inhibitors (rivaroxaban, apixaban, and edoxaban) and direct thrombin inhibitors (dabigatran). Direct factor Xa inhibitors work by preventing factor Xa from cleaving prothrombin into its active form, thrombin, and thus blocking the coagulation cascade. Direct thrombin inhibitors instead bind directly to thrombin and inhibit activity in both free and fibrin-bound thrombin. DOACs are metabolised in the liver and partially excreted by the kidneys to varying degrees.

DOACs have been found to be non-inferior to warfarin in studies in both venous thromboembolism (VTE) recurrence and bleeding risk. To date, there are no head-to-head studies comparing efficacy between DOACs; however, apixaban and rivaroxaban compared to the other DOACs appears to have the least major bleeding risk. Additionally, apixaban and rivaroxaban can be started without needing to be concurrently

Table 3. A list of the most used DOACs. There are two DOAC subclasses: Direct factor Xa inhibitors (rivaroxaban, apixaban, and edoxaban) and direct thrombin inhibitors (dabigatran). All DOACs are oral agents with either daily or twice daily dosing. DOACs have a rapid onset/offset, does not require routine monitoring, metabolise in the liver and renally cleared. Only dabigatran can be dialysed Prothrombin complex concentrate products (PCC) and activated charcoal as reversal agent for all DOACs. Reversal agents are available for rivaroxaban and apixaban (andexanet alfa) and dabigatran (idarucizumab).

	Direct factor Xa inhibitors			Direct thrombin inhibitors
Drug Name	**Rivaroxaban**	**Apixaban**	**Edoxaban**	**Dabigatran**
Dosing	15 mg by mouth twice daily for 21 days, followed by 20 mg once daily	10 mg by mouth twice daily for 7 days, followed by 5 mg twice daily	Start concurrently with parenteral heparin for 5 days, then 60 mg daily	Start concurrently with parenteral heparin for 5 days, then 150 mg twice daily
Reversal agents	Activated charcoal if ingested <2 hours			
	Andexanet alfa			Idarucizumab
	4-factor PCC			Activate PCC
Dialyzable	No			Yes
Monitoring	Anti-factor Xa levels analysis is available, but not routinely monitored			Diluted thrombin time
Onset	2.5–4 hours	3–4 hours	1–2 hours	1–2 hours
Half-life	5–13 hours	~12 hours	10–14 hours	12–28 hours
Metabolism	Hepatic			
Renal clearance	35%	27%	50%	80%
Special considerations	May have lower bleeding risk			

bridged with parenteral heparin or enoxaparin due to their rapid onset, making them a convenient and safe option for PE patients. Initiation of dabigatran and edoxaban require concurrently dosing with parenteral heparin for 5 days following PE, making them less desirable than their counterparts.

While laboratory assays exist to evaluate DOAC levels, there is no utility in routine monitoring. In clinical practice, anti-factor Xa levels and diluted thrombin time (dTT) assays are usually done in the context of subtherapeutic levels suspicion and concerns of treatment failure. Though these assays exist they may not be readily available everywhere and no universal guidelines exist to correlate results to therapeutic efficacy.

For a long time one of the major drawbacks of DOACs was their lack of reversal agents for life-threatening bleeding. PCC products are effective reversal agents, but their onset of action is slow. To date, there are two reversal agents available for DOACs: andexanet alfa (rivaroxaban and apixaban) and idarucizumab (dabigatran). Andexanet alfa is a highly effective recombinant modified Factor Xa protein that can rapidly neutralise anti-factor Xa activity within minutes. Idarucizumab is an antibody derived non-competitive inhibitor to dabigatran and rapidly reduces its affinity for thrombin.

Indirect thrombin inhibitors

Indirect thrombin inhibitors are not considered first line options in most PE situations. The most used indirect thrombin inhibitor is enoxaparin. Enoxaparin is a low molecular weight heparin (LMWH) and is only available as a subcutaneous injection. Enoxaparin works by inhibiting antithrombin III activity resulting in significant factor Xa activity inhibition. Unlike unfractionated heparin, enoxaparin has little impact on the partial thromboplastin time (PTT), thus PTT monitoring is not recommended.

Enoxaparin is commonly used to treat PE in pregnant women, patients with active malignancy, and as bridging prior to procedures. Enoxaparin does not cross the placenta and is the safest anticoagulation option in pregnancy. In patients with active malignancy, enoxaparin has been the first choice due to its lower risk of bleeding and rates of PE recurrence. Additionally, enoxaparin is commonly used to bridge DOACs prior to planned surgery or procedures to minimised bleeding and clotting risk for patients who cannot come off anticoagulation.

Indirect factor Xa inhibitors

Indirect factor Xa inhibitors are the least used anticoagulant class for the treatment of PE. Fondaparinux is the only anticoagulant in this class and is available as a subcutaneous injection. Fondaparinux is a synthetic derivative pentasaccharide that inhibits antithrombin III and selectively inhibits factor Xa activity. Fondaparinux has a longer half-life than other LMWH and it can be used in patients with a history of heparin-induced thrombocytopenia (HIT). Generally, fondaparinux is the most expensive option and is only considered in the setting of recurrent PEs due to anti-coagulant therapy failures.

Selecting the Most Appropriate Anticoagulant for Your Patient

When selecting an anticoagulant, it is important to ask yourself the following questions:

- Are there any identifiable PE risk factor(s) that I must consider?
- Does my patient have comorbidities that would affect the pharmacokinetic of the selected anticoagulant?
- Are there any socioeconomic barriers that will impact my patient's compliance to the selected therapy?

In the majority of PE cases, after thoroughly reviewing the patient's clinical chart and identifying any patient-related barriers, the anticoagulants of choice usually narrow down to either apixaban or rivaroxaban. Apixaban and rivaroxaban are the best options due to their rapid onset, simple oral dosing regimen, lower bleeding profile among the DOACs and their similar therapeutic efficacy to warfarin without the complicated dose titration and monitoring.

In conditions where apixaban and rivaroxaban are contraindicated, warfarin is a good alternative. Enoxaparin can be considered in specific situations as an alternative, but cost and subcutaneous administration is not ideal for most patients. Edoxaban, dabigatran, and fondaparinux are not commonly used unless an alternative anticoagulant is warranted, due to treatment failure.

While warfarin is usually the least expensive outpatient anticoagulation option, it is important to acknowledge that it requires frequent monitoring and compliance on the part of the patient. Discuss with the patient their social situation and evaluate how realistic it is for them to be able to adhere to frequent monitoring visits and laboratory blood tests. Consider access to transportation, diet, medical literacy, and willingness to adhere to monitoring regimen as these can affect patient outcomes. If a patient gets lost to follow up it will become likely they will end up sub- or supra-therapeutic with risk of clotting or bleeding, respectively. In patients who can adhere to monitoring requirements, warfarin is a cost-effective option with once daily dosing.

One of the leading factors to medication noncompliance and ultimately treatment failure in those receiving care under insurance is high out-of-pocket expense of anticoagulation therapy. From the beginning, it is important to work with the patient, their insurance, and outpatient pharmacy to find the most cost-effective option. DOACs tend to have a high co-pay cost, but due to their lack of routine monitoring parameters the cumulative cost over time may likely be equivalent to that of VKAs and its monitoring cost. For some patients, the higher upfront cost of DOACs may not be feasible and warfarin is the cheapest option.

Anticoagulant preference in specific patient populations

In specific patient populations (Table 4), selecting an inappropriate anticoagulant therapy could result in subtherapeutic levels and dramatically increase their risk of recurrence or supratherapeutic levels and significantly increase their bleeding risk.

- *Patients with moderate to severe hepatic impairment*: DOACs are not recommended due to concerns of inconsistency in DOAC dose levels. Warfarin is the treatment of choice.
- *Patients with chronic renal disease*: DOACs are not recommended due to concerns of inconsistency in DOAC dose levels. Warfarin is another good choice here.
- *Patients with active malignancy*: There are supporting studies demonstrating apixaban as good alternatives to enoxaparin. However, DOACs should still be used with caution in cancer patients due to higher bleeding risk compared to enoxaparin.
- *Pregnancy*: DOACs are not recommended in pregnant patients due to lack of supporting clinical data and observation suggests DOACs can cross the placenta. Additionally, warfarin can have teratogenic effects

on the foetus, hence enoxaparin is the only safe treatment option during pregnancy.

- *Antiphospholipid syndrome*: Warfarin is the only anticoagulant recommended, due to increased bleeding risk with the other anticoagulant classes. Due to higher PE recurrence rates, recommended INR is usually >2.5.
- *Morbidly obese patients*: Besides apixaban, most DOACs are not recommended in, due to concerns for subtherapeutic level. The treatments of choice are warfarin and enoxaparin.

Table 4. Summary of anticoagulant preference in specific patient populations. In most PE cases, either apixaban or rivaroxaban are considered first-line treatment options. In specific conditions, VKAs and indirect thrombin inhibitors are the preferred anticoagulants. DOACs are not recommended in specific hepatic disease, renal disease, pregnancy, gastrointestinal absorption issues, and antiphospholipid syndrome.

	Direct factor Xa inhibitors	Direct thrombin inhibitors	Indirect/direct thrombin inhibitors	Vitamin K antagonists
Moderate to severe liver disease	Not recommended, unknown efficacy		Yes, alternative option, but close monitoring	Treatment of choice
Chronic renal disease (GFR <30)			Yes, enoxaparin only	
Active malignancy	Apixaban Use with caution	Not recommended, may increase bleeding	Yes, enoxaparin	Not recommended, may increase bleeding
Pregnancy	Not recommended, crosses placenta			Not recommended, teratogenic effects
Antiphospholipid syndrome	Not recommended, may increase bleeding			Treatment of choice
Obesity (BMI >40)	Apixaban, use with caution	Not recommended, unknown efficacy	Yes, enoxaparin as alternative	

Important Counselling Points

Once you and your patient have decided on anticoagulant therapy, the next critical step is to counsel them on the following:

- Emphasise the importance of medication compliance to reduce their risks of clinical worsening, bleeding, and recurrence risk.
- While on anticoagulation, it is normal to experience longer than normal bleeding time before haemostasis is achieved and it is normal to see bruising on the extremities while on anticoagulation.
- Review the risk of major bleeding and the importance of avoiding activities with high risk of serious head trauma or injury such as contact sports and high-risk activities.
- For planned procedures or surgeries, it is important to discuss anticoagulation plans to minimise their procedural-related bleeding risks.
- For females of childbearing age, counselling them on the risk of any teratogenic effects or fetal harm. Additionally, it is important to mention to them the risk of heavier bleeding during their menstrual cycles.

For all patients who end up on prolonged anticoagulation treatment, it is important to have ongoing conversations regarding the bleeding risk, benefits of anticoagulation, any new social or economic barriers to treatment. Additionally, periodically patients should be reevaluated for consideration of anticoagulation dose reduction or discontinuation.

For How Long?

In clinical practice, once the patient starts anticoagulant therapy, the next challenging decision is to determine the proper treatment duration. The main goal of anticoagulation therapy is to reduce the PE recurrence risk. There are certain identifiable risk factors and associated comorbidities that may influence the recurrence risk (Table 5). By categorising a risk factor as reversible, acquired, or heritable, this will assist you in risk stratifying your patient's recurrence risk and aid in determining the most appropriate treatment duration.

PE due to transient or reversible risk factors (i.e., surgery, hospitalisation, hormonal therapy, smoking or pregnancy) tends to have a lower rate of recurrence compared to the others. Patients should be anticoagulated for a minimum of 3 months and then reevaluated to

Table 5. A list of common PE risk factors and their treatment duration. PE risk factors are categorised into transient (reversible), acquired or heritable risk factors. Risk factors can influence the treatment duration.

PE risk factors
Transient or reversible factors (treatment duration 3–6 months)
• Surgery or trauma within the last 3 months
• Hospitalisation or immobility ≥3 days
• Pregnancy
• Hormone replacement therapy
• Oral contraception
• Smoking/nicotine products
Acquired factors (treatment duration >6 months)
• Advanced age
• Obesity
• Chronic diseases
• Active malignancy
Heritable factors (treatment duration >6 months — indefinitely)
• Thrombophilias
• Coagulation disorders

determine whether prolonged anticoagulation is needed. For most of these PE cases, usually 3 months of anticoagulation is appropriate if the transient factor has been addressed or reversed. Follow-up chest imaging and echocardiogram should be completed to assist in determining whether appropriateness of prolonged anticoagulation therapy and whether further evaluation is warranted to rule out chronic thromboembolic conditions, such as chronic thromboembolic pulmonary hypertension (CTEPH).

The PE recurrence risk is more unpredictable for patients whose PE is due to an acquired risk factor (i.e., obesity and cardiac disease and active malignancy). These patients tend to have multiple risk factors and thus increase their PE recurrence risk. Most of these patients are usually on prolonged anticoagulation courses >6 months and in some instances such as active malignancy, it can be indefinitely or until the malignancy is in remission. Additionally, these patients may have a higher risk of treatment failure, therefore, close monitoring and expert referral for further management is encouraged.

Patients with heritable risk factors (i.e., thrombophilia and coagulability disorders), recurrent PEs, CTEPH and unidentifiable risk factors have the highest risk of recurrence and therefore are usually on indefinite anti-coagulant therapy. However, it is important to periodically reevaluate the risk and benefits of long-term anticoagulation as well as considerations of lower the anticoagulant dose with treatment durations beyond 6 months.

Conclusion

With advances in the field of post-acute PE management and prevention, the treatment paradigm has shifted away from VKAs as the treatment of choice to DOACs, specifically, apixaban and rivaroxaban. This practice shift has simplified the outpatient PE management algorithm to orally administered agents with rapid onsets and without the need for complicated dosing titrations and consistent monitoring. VKAs and LMWH still have their place in select patient populations where DOACs are contraindicated or if there are pharmacokinetic efficacy concerns.

Treatment duration is based on reducing the risk of PE recurrence. Transient and reversible risk factors have the lowest PE recurrence rate and the most predictable anticoagulant treatment regimen. Conversely, determining the best treatment duration may be challenging in patients with multiple PE risk factors and underlying chronic morbidities. Many of these patients end up on prolong or lifelong anticoagulant therapy due to their high PE recurrence risk.

For all patients, after prolonged anticoagulation therapy, it is reasonable to consider anticoagulant therapy dose reduction or discontinuation. However, if at any point after dose reduction or anticoagulation discontinuation, they developed another PE, then lifelong anticoagulation is warranted.

Bibliography

Agnelli, G. *et al.* (2020). Apixaban for the treatment of venous thromboembolism associated with cancer, *The New England Journal of Medicine*, 382, pp. 1599–1607.

Cohen *et al.* (2021). Effectiveness and safety of apixaban vs. warfarin in venous thromboembolism patients with obesity and morbid obesity, *Journal of Clinical Medicine*, 10(2), pp. 200.

Dawwas, G.K., Brown, J., Dietrich, E., and Park, H. (2019). Effectiveness and safety of apixaban versus rivaroxaban for prevention of recurrent venous thromboembolism and adverse bleeding events in patients with venous thromboembolism: A retrospective population-based cohort analysis, *Lancet Haematology*, 6(1), pp. e20–e28.

Konstantinides *et al.* (2020). ESC Scientific Document Group, 2019 ESC Guidelines for the diagnosis and management of acute pulmonary embolism developed in collaboration with the European Respiratory Society (ERS): The Task Force for the diagnosis and management of acute pulmonary embolism of the European Society of Cardiology (ESC), *European Heart Journal*, 4(4), pp. 543–603.

O'Reilly, R.A. and Aggeler, P.M. (1968). Studies on coumarin anticoagulant drugs. Initiation of warfarin therapy without a loading dose, *Circulation*, 38(1), pp. 169–177.

Ortel *et al.* (2020). American Society of Hematology 2020 guidelines for management of venous thromboembolism: Treatment of deep vein thrombosis and pulmonary embolism, *Blood Advances,* 4(19), pp. 4693–4738.

Van Es, N., Coppens, M., Schulman, S., Middeldorp, S., and Büller, H.R. (2014). Direct oral anticoagulants compared with vitamin K antagonists for acute venous thromboembolism: Evidence from phase 3 trials, *Blood*, 18, 124(12), pp. 1968–1975.

https://doi.org/10.1142/9781800612778_0014

Chapter 14

Follow-Up Assessment — Who to Follow and How to Investigate?

Luke Howard* and Colm McCabe†

**Department of Cardiology, Imperial College Healthcare
NHS Trust, UK*

*†Royal Brompton and Harefield Hospitals, Guy's and
St Thomas' NHS Foundation Trust, London, UK*

Abstract

The follow up of acute pulmonary embolism presents a growing challenge to clinicians with decisions involving anticoagulation management, screening for complications, and investigations around persistent breathlessness key to patient recovery. Inconsistency in approach to clinical management in this setting is perhaps an inevitable consequence of a rapidly evolving evidence base for therapeutic anticoagulation options involving treatment dose and duration as well as an increased awareness of chronic thromboembolic pulmonary hypertension, a rare but severe long-term complication of pulmonary embolism. Here we review suggested clinical approaches to the investigation of patients diagnosed with pulmonary embolism focusing on the investigation of persistently symptomatic patients at risk of chronic complications. Additional discussion is provided on topical aspects of chronic thromboembolic disease less incorporated in guidelines concerning pulmonary embolism follow up.

Introduction

The clinical follow up of patients presenting with acute pulmonary embolism (PE) remains highly variable with no consensus on optimal strategy. This applies especially to patients experiencing persistent dyspnoea despite a minimum of 3 months anticoagulation, now the standard of care for all patients diagnosed with acute PE. The variation in PE follow-up strategy stems from several factors including front-door clinical evaluation by clinicians of multiple specialty background, differing availability of local services including ambulatory care to facilitate rapid outpatient review, variable interpretation of risk of PE recurrence, and continuing uncertainty over how to screen for long-term PE complications. More fundamentally, the low number of prospective studies testing specific follow-up strategies in PE follow up has meant recent guideline recommendations are largely based on expert opinion.

In the patient demonstrating complete functional recovery after acute PE with anticoagulation therapy alone, the dose and duration of anticoagulation may in the vast majority be determined by the presence or absence of predisposing risk factors at diagnosis (Chapter 13, Table 5). In contrast, patients in whom functional recovery is somehow incomplete despite adherence to therapeutic anticoagulation require an alternative approach that extends beyond anticoagulation management. This chapter primarily focuses on the second patient group in whom the diagnosis of long-term PE complications carries greater relevance. Typically, these patients complain of persistent dyspnoea or chest discomfort with impaired quality of life compared to pre-morbid levels. These patients represent a growing burden on healthcare resources with a higher requirement for psychosocial support, greater likelihood of impaired exercise tolerance, and increasing eligibility for exercise rehabilitation programs.

Why Follow-Up Patients with Acute PE?

The follow up of PE serves numerous purposes including the identification and management of bleeding on anticoagulation, assessment and screening for malignancy and thrombophilia, and evaluation of patients for signs of incomplete functional recovery. An increasing trend towards early review around 2–4 weeks after diagnosis offers the opportunity to review and confirm the diagnosis, address anticoagulation compliance, re-check relevant drug interactions, identify occult bleeding, and where relevant, complete age-specific malignancy screening. At 3 months, follow up serves more to direct long-term anticoagulation management and stratify the investigation of potential long-term complications. This "dual assessment" approach to follow-up carries significant advantages for anticoagulation management and screening. However, in the authors' view, in patients with smaller subsegmental PEs adequately risk stratified for risk of recurrence at diagnosis and where compliance and duration of anticoagulation have been already safely assessed at diagnosis, follow up may not always be required.

At 3–6 months following PE, several large patient series suggest that in up to 60% of patients diagnosed with acute PE, recovery to premorbid levels of function is incomplete despite anticoagulation. This may be predicted by an increased age at diagnosis, the presence of cardiac or pulmonary comorbidity, higher BMI, smoking status, higher pulmonary pressures, right ventricular dysfunction at presentation and evidence of residual pulmonary vascular obstruction at follow up. Historical scintigraphy studies evaluating recovery after PE have demonstrated a lack of association between functional recovery and normalisation of perfusion after acute PE. This can give rise to uncertainty over the requirement for continued anticoagulation where persistent perfusion abnormalities coexist with exercise intolerance. We know from the ELOPE study, a prospective Canadian study of 100 patients followed to determine functional recovery after acute PE, that post-PE breathlessness relates poorly to both choice of anticoagulation and the degree of thrombotic obstruction. However, the comparatively low burden of thrombus seen in this study means that questions remain around the optimal anticoagulation strategy in patients who may demonstrate larger thrombotic burdens at follow up. However, much needed evidence is beginning to emerge which may help guide treatment in this area.

Central to the evaluation of patients with persistent symptoms after PE are investigations directed towards the early diagnosis of chronic thromboembolic pulmonary hypertension (CTEPH). CTEPH is the gravest long-term complication of acute PE and is characterised by endothelialisation of thrombus, vascular web formation, chronic fibrosis and vascular remodelling in the distal pulmonary arteries. The incidence of CTEPH after acute PE is unknown with studies suggesting a range between 0.4% and 4%. Although less than 30% of patients diagnosed with CTEPH report a diagnosis of previous PE, it seems the condition may also evolve from a succession of smaller "subclinical" thrombotic insults which trigger a secondary pulmonary vasculopathy. The diagnosis of CTEPH requires demonstration of pulmonary hypertension at right heart catheterisation (currently defined by a mean pulmonary artery pressure ≥25 mmHg), in the presence of persistent perfusion defects on V/Q scintigraphy following at least 3 months therapeutic anticoagulation. Recent proposals to reduce the mean PA pressure threshold from ≥25 to >20 mmHg in pulmonary hypertension have not yet been adopted in CTEPH.

The recently reported multicentre Inshape II study prospectively validated a CTEPH "prediction tool" using a PE follow-up algorithm in over 400 patients. Based on the absence of ECG criteria of RV hypertrophy and abnormal NT-proBNP levels employed as CTEPH "rule-out" criteria, CTEPH could be accurately excluded without requirement for echocardiography at follow up in 10 out of 13 (77%) of patients ultimately diagnosed with CTEPH. A further recently reported prospective multicentre study of over 1000 patients with acute PE in Germany (FOCUS) followed for a median of 732 days showed an estimated cumulative incidence of CTEPH of 2.3%. Post-PE impairment evaluated by standardised criteria was evident in 16% of patients who also emerged with higher risk of re-hospitalisation and death as well as worse quality of life.

Chronic thromboembolic pulmonary disease (CTEPD), as well as CTEPH, is also haemodynamically defined by right heart catheterisation criteria. CTEPD has come to include patients with evidence of pulmonary vascular obstruction as well as a mean pulmonary artery pressure <25 mmHg at rest assessed by right heart catheterisation. The redefining of pulmonary hypertension to a pressure of >20 mmHg, would in practice convert some patients from a diagnosis of CTEPD to CTEPH, although the pulmonary vascular resistance (PVR) threshold of ≥3 Wood Units may not always be met. The literature on CTEPD supports an abnormal pulmonary vascular response to exercise in this patient group and just as with CTEPH, its diagnosis is usually only confirmed after at least 3 months anticoagulation. In recent years, the term post-PE syndrome has also emerged as an extrapolation from the "post-thrombotic syndrome" associated with long-term complications of DVT. Post-PE syndrome not only includes patients with CTEPH and CTEPD but also those where a pathophysiological link between previous PE and symptoms is suspected. While the definition of CTEPH remains robust, imaging and physiological criteria that discriminate patients with CTEPD and those with post-PE breathlessness of unrelated cause are currently lacking. Refinement of the definition of CTEPD that considers the extent and heterogeneity of pulmonary vascular obstruction along with secondary effects on RV function will be key.

Screening for malignancy and thrombophilia

A VTE diagnosis confers an up to six-fold risk of malignancy compared to age and sex-matched controls with the highest risk in those over 50 who are within 6 months of diagnosis of an unprovoked VTE event. Specific screening should be guided by local and national guidelines but may be based largely around elements listed in Table 1. Extensive CT contrast imaging of the chest and abdomen and 18-fluorodeoxyglucose Positron Emission Tomography CT have been shown to identify more cancer diagnoses around the time of the VTE episode; however, earlier detection has not yet translated into an increased survival benefit.

Up to 30% of patients with VTE harbour an inherited thrombophilia, however testing is recommended in two specific settings:

(1) Where the result is expected to modify the dose, duration, or type of anticoagulant.
(2) Where there are implications around pregnancy counselling in female first-degree relatives.

The presence of inherited thrombophilia in a patient at increased risk of VTE recurrence in whom anticoagulation discontinuation is being considered may potentially direct clinicians towards prescription of long-term anticoagulation. Screening for the presence of antiphospholipid antibodies

Table 1. Available screening tools used to evaluate malignancy potential around a diagnosis of acute PE.

Recommended routine investigations	More extensive investigations with unclear benefit
• Physical examination	• Abdominopelvic CT + mammography in women
• Chest X-ray	
• Full blood count, serum calcium, and liver function tests	• 18F — PET CT
	• Tumour marker profile
• Urinalysis	

is currently only recommended for patients with clinically suspicious features such as a history of arterial thrombosis, prior thrombosis at unusual sites, a history of recurrent miscarriage or pre-eclampsia/eclampsia, auto-immune disease, younger age at diagnosis, or patients with a previously unexplained elevation in APTT levels prior to anticoagulation. However, contemporary literature on the down-titration of DOAC dose at 6 months from PE diagnosis has meant more widespread screening for antiphospholipid antibody syndrome (APLS) is often clinically helpful, as this approach is contraindicated in those with APLS this condition. This is especially true for patients identified to have "double" or "triple-positive" APLS by laboratory criteria (Chapter 11, Table 1), which would ordinarily prompt a switch to Vitamin K antagonist-based anticoagulation.

What to Assess at a Follow-Up Visit 3–6 Months after PE

The recent ESC/ERS guidelines in acute PE stress that after 3–6 months anti-coagulation, no patients should be lost to follow-up and all should be assessed for persisting or new-onset dyspnoea or functional limitation. If present, a staged diagnostic workup should be initiated to exclude CTEPH or CTEPD, and to detect/treat comorbidity or "simple" deconditioning. At this visit, all patients including those reporting complete recovery, should undergo a clinical evaluation which as a minimum may include the following investigations:

- SpO_2, systemic BP, heart rate measurement
- 12-lead ECG
- FBC, U&Es, LFTs, Iron profile, anti-Cardiolipin Ab, anti-β-2 glycoprotein level, lupus anticoagulant (if not performed already)

Typically, in up to one half of cases, patients report complete resolution of symptoms. If screening for malignancy, assessment of bleeding risk and anticoagulation duration is already determined, the patient may be reassured and discharged from follow up. Follow-up imaging is not recommended in asymptomatic patients, although it may be considered in patients with risk factors for development of CTEPH (Table 2) as not all CTEPH may present within 3 months of an incident PE.

In the persistently symptomatic patient, consideration should be given to the likelihood of PE recurrence, unresolved thrombotic obstruction

Table 2.   Risk factors for CTEPH.

Present at diagnosis	Assessed at 3–6 months follow-up
• Recurrent, unprovoked, or idiopathic PE • Large perfusion defects when PE was detected • Younger or older age when PE was detected • Pulmonary-artery systolic pressure >50 mm Hg at first manifestation of PE • Persistent pulmonary hypertension (PH) evident when echocardiography is performed 6 months after acute PE was detected • Imaging features of CTEPH on presenting CTPA	• Ventriculo-arterial shunts • Prior infection IV lines or pacemaker • Prior splenectomy • Non-O blood group • Thrombophilia esp. Antiphospholipid Antibody Syndrome

(CTEPD or CTEPH) or the emergence of alternative pathology. Clinical evaluation should include cardiovascular and respiratory examination directed at identification of right ventricular compromise and pulmonary hypertension. Cardiac evaluation may reveal elevated venous pressures, a loud pulmonary S2, and prominent hepatojugular reflex. Peripheral oedema or ascites may also be seen in advanced cases with or without low systemic oxygen saturation levels.

Echocardiography is key in this setting with the risk of pulmonary hypertension determined by a doppler envelope tricuspid regurgitant jet velocity >2.8 m/s. Guidelines for acute PE management have further partitioned the likelihood of CTEPH into low, intermediate, and high probability of pulmonary hypertension with further investigation including measurement of serum NT-pro BNP levels, assessment of CTEPH risk factors, and where feasible, identification of specific echocardiographic findings and cardiopulmonary exercise test outcomes (Table 3). In patients with an intermediate or high probability of pulmonary hypertension based on echocardiography, the suggested first-line imaging modality in symptomatic patients following PE is V/Q scintigraphy to evaluate for CTEPH, however other modalities may be suitable, especially with the advent of iodine mapping on dual-energy CT where local expertise may differ.

The flowchart in Figure 1 includes a suggested pathway for investigating patients with persistent dyspnoea following acute PE providing additional context around the investigation of patients with a low risk of

Table 3.   Indicators of CTEPH at follow up (consider diagnosis if ≥1 factor present).

Echocardiography	• Enlarged RV, increased RV/LV ratio >1.0
	• Flattened interventricular septum (parasternal short axis view)
	• Distended IVC with reduced collapse on inspiration
	• Pulmonary acceleration time <60 md, or mid-systolic notch in pulmonary ejection envelope
	• Right heart thrombus
	• TAPSE <16 mm
	• RV S' velocity Tricuspid valve annulus <9.5 m/s
Cardiopulmonary exercise testing	• Reduced peak VO_2
	• Increased VE/VCO_2 slope >35
	• Reduced end tidal CO_2
	• Increased Vd/Vt (requires ABG analysis)
Laboratory testing	• Elevated NT-pro BNP

CTEPH at follow-up assessment. It should be stressed that this approach has not been subject to evaluation in management studies but instead offers a simplified approach providing differentiation between CTEPD and post-PE breathlessness at 3–6 months by sole reliance on imaging. The need for cardiopulmonary exercise testing (CPET) which carries greater variability in interpretation is de-emphasised and so may be deferred to specialist centre evaluation.

What Alternative Diagnoses Should I Consider in Post-PE Breathlessness?

As PE represents a common complication of several cardiopulmonary disorders, interpretation of investigations relating to persistent dyspnoea must therefore account for the contribution from any pre-existent pathology. Where CTEPH or CTEPD fail to account for symptoms, three prevalent conditions contributing to post-PE breathlessness include deconditioning, dysfunctional breathing, and in rare circumstances, the development of autonomic dysfunction. While a complete review of these is beyond the scope of this chapter, diagnostic considerations are included in the following for section further guidance. Table 4 outlines the principle identifiers of each condition on cardiopulmonary exercise testing.

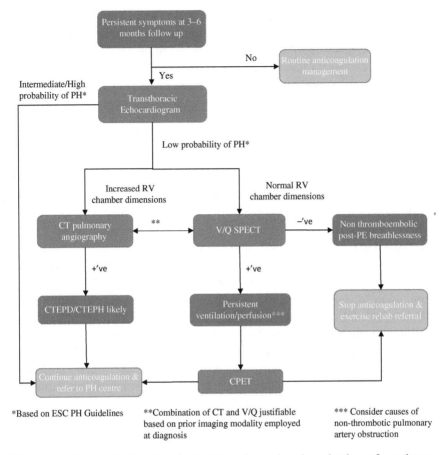

Figure 1. Proposed algorithm to facilitate image-based evaluation of persistent symptoms in patients following PE.

Deconditioning

The development of deconditioning following acute PE is probably the most common cause of exercise limitation following acute PE. Deconditioning may be suspected clinically by recent weight gain and a sedentary lifestyle. In more athletic individuals, unaccustomed inactivity may bring about detraining making its diagnosis harder. The formal assessment of deconditioning relies on the demonstration of an abnormally low anaerobic threshold (<50% predicted VO_2 max) measured during a symptom-limited incremental ramp CPET in tandem with associated features of impaired cardiovascular adaptation on exercise. Its diagnosis also relies on the absence of features of other cardiorespiratory pathology on exercise such that in many ways, deconditioning remains a diagnosis of exclusion. Its treatment requires a proactive approach engaging physiotherapy and rehabilitation programs and, where feasible, weight reduction.

Dysfunctional breathing

Dysfunctional breathing is an umbrella term for a variety of conditions in which an irregular breathing pattern, at rest or during exercise, gives rise to breathlessness. It is characterised by a lack of organic respiratory disease or a level of breathlessness felt to be disproportionate to the extent of underlying organic disease. Dysfunctional breathing outside the context of PE may be present in up to 10% of the population with an increased prevalence in asthma. Although there is no consensus on its exact definition, recent proposals include its subdivision into hyperventilation syndrome, periodic dead sigh breathing, thoracic dominant breathing, forced abdominal expiration, and thoraco-abdominal expiration. This categorisation was intended to supplant both the thoracic and extra-thoracic classification of dysfunctional breathing and structural and functional forms previously in use. Its development following PE remains incompletely understood and frequently it may overlap with other comorbidities.

Table 4.   CPET evaluation during PE follow up.

Conditions contributing to post PE breathlessness — Features on CPET	
Deconditioning	• Reduced peak VO_2 (<80% predicted)
	• Reduced anaerobic threshold (<50% predicted VO_2 max)
	• Elevated HR/VO_2 slope
	• Normal VO_2/work rate slope (~10 mL/min/Watt)
	• Absent features of cardiovascular impairment
	• Normal ECG
Dysfunctional breathing	• Variable breath by breath tidal volume excursion in early to moderate exercise
	• Mildly elevated VE/VCO_2 slope (28–35)
	• Low end-tidal pCO_2 if coexistent hyperventilation
Autonomic dysfunction	• Low peak oxygen pulse (<80% predicted)
	• Elevated HR response to exercise

Autonomic dysfunction

A very limited number of patients suffers exercise limitation of more obscure origin following PE. Of these, disordered autonomic control of the cardiovascular system may contribute to symptom limitation particularly after PEs of large thrombotic burden. Affected patients may demonstrate an increased chronotropic response to exercise, postural haemodynamic instability, and associated breathing pattern response not unlike mild hyperventilation. Clinical features are analogous to postural orthostatic tachycardia syndrome (POTS) and orthostatic hypotension, however, a pathophysiological link between acute PE and dysautonomia remains unproven.

Points of Contention

Direct oral anticoagulants (DOACs) now offer a simplified anticoagulation regimen for the treatment of all venous thromboembolism (VTE) and in several landmark studies have demonstrated non-inferiority to Vitamin K antagonists in amelioration of risk of VTE recurrence with reduced rates of anticoagulation-associated bleeding. The additional possibility of de-escalation in the dose of Rivaroxaban or Apixaban at 6 months which confers a reduced risk of VTE recurrence with improved rates of anticoagulation-associated bleeding has further tipped the balance in favour of use of DOACs over coumarin-based anticoagulants. It is noteworthy however that in these studies, which were not exclusive to PE, "clinical equipoise" was employed as eligibility criteria to randomise patients to full or half-dose anticoagulation. Persistence of symptoms across PE and deep vein thrombosis (DVT) during follow up may be clinically relevant to anticoagulation duration as the landscape of prevention of long-term VTE complications may differ between DVT and PE. In particular, whereas catheter-based clot dispersion techniques carry established evidence in the acute phase of DVT treatment, catheter-based intervention at diagnosis of PE is comparatively less robust with little data on its long-term effect on symptom recovery.

The importance of appropriate long-term anticoagulation in PE has been underscored in recent ESC PE guidelines especially in cases of unprovoked PE. Of the multiple contributors to breathlessness at PE follow up, CTEPD has in recent years emerged as an indication for anticoagulation without the backing of substantial evidence. Early distinction between CTEPD and CTEPH is usually feasible at a 3 month follow-up review.

However, the lack of data supporting requirement for long-term anticoagulation in CTEPD with additional uncertainty over what degree of clot burden may be "required" to fulfil a diagnosis of CTEPD suggested by V/Q or CTPA, means the decision to continue anticoagulation may not be straightforward. This choice may be further complicated where CTEPD has developed following an acute PE associated with major transient risk factors (see Chapter 13, Table 5), such as immobilisation or recent major surgery where anticoagulation may be ordinarily discontinued at 3 months.

A diagnostic label of CTEPD also remains too broad to allow development of robust guidelines on the management of CTEPD, which includes the question of anticoagulation duration. A diagnosis of CTEPD may in future be better reserved for patients with persistent symptoms in whom the amount of residual proximal thrombus on CTPA would prompt potential consideration of surgical referral for pulmonary endarterectomy, the gold standard surgical treatment for CTEPH. Patients with CTEPD and these diagnostic features commonly demonstrate mild dilatation of the right ventricle on echocardiogram, despite low risk features for pulmonary hypertension, which is in contrast to patients with smaller perfusion deficits in whom right ventricular appearances are frequently within normal limits. Using this distinction, patients with a large thrombotic burden on CT angiography would be prioritised to prolonged anticoagulation irrespective of PE risk factors at presentation.

It is notable here that in the long-term studies of DOAC continuation beyond 6 months, where clinicians were in equipoise over whether to stop anticoagulation, no distinction was made between patients with and without symptoms. With few individuals diagnosed with CTEPD eligible for PEA, anticoagulation is likely to remain the only therapy offered to most patients. Diagnostic criteria that best define those likely to benefit from long-term anticoagulation from those in whom anticoagulation may be safely discontinued without detriment to quality of life or risk of PE recurrence, are clearly needed although a future haemodynamic redefinition of CTEPH which may or may not include a PVR threshold would admittedly change this landscape again.

Summary

A recent ESC/ERS position paper has issued a "call to action" towards a holistic approach to PE care. Physicians in this arena are charged with complex assessments ranging from acute care aspects of anticoagulation management and risk assessment for PE recurrence to life-long management of PE complications and impairment in quality of life. Emergence of the post-PE syndrome has brought previously disregarded aspects of management such as cardiac rehabilitation to the forefront of care. At a time when front door PE care is witnessing rapid changes in practice, the comprehensive follow-up assessment of PE must attract equal attention.

Bibliography

Boon, G.J.A.M., Ende-Verhaar, Y.M., Bavalia, R., El Bouazzaoui, L.H., Delcroix, M., Dzikowska-Diduch, O., Huisman, M.V., Kurnicka, K., Mairuhu, A.T.A., Middeldorp, S., Pruszczyk, P., Ruigrok, D., Verhamme, P., Vliegen, H.W., Vonk Noordegraaf, A., Vriend, J.W.J., and Klok, F.A. (2021). InShape II study group. Non-invasive early exclusion of chronic thromboembolic pulmonary hypertension after acute pulmonary embolism: The InShape II study, *Thorax*, 76(10), pp. 1002–1009.

Enden, T., Haig, Y., Kløw, N.E., Slagsvold, C.E., Sandvik, L., Ghanima, W., Hafsahl, G., Holme, P.A., Holmen, L.O., Njaastad, A.M., Sandbæk, G., Sandset, P.M., and CaVenT Study Group (2012). Long-term outcome after additional catheter-directed thrombolysis versus standard treatment for acute iliofemoral deep vein thrombosis (the CaVenT study): A randomised controlled trial, *Lancet*, 379(9810), pp. 31–38.

Howard, L.S. (2018). Non-vitamin K antagonist oral anticoagulants for pulmonary embolism: Who, where and for how long? *Expert Review of Respiratory Medicine*, 12(5), pp. 387–402.

Kahn, S.R., Hirsch, A.M., Akaberi, A., Hernandez, P., Anderson, D.R., Wells, P.S., Rodger, M.A., Solymoss, S., Kovacs, M.J., Rudski, L., Shimony, A., Dennie, C., Rush, C., Geerts, W.H., Aaron, S.D., and Granton, J.T. (2017). Functional and exercise limitations after a first episode of pulmonary embolism: Results of the ELOPE prospective cohort study, *Chest*, 151(5), pp. 1058–1068.

Klok, F.A., Ageno, W., Ay, C., Bäck, M., Barco, S., Bertoletti, L., Becattini, C., Carlsen, J., Delcroix, M., van Es, N., Huisman, M.V,, Jara-Palomares, L., Konstantinides, S., Lang, I., Meyer, G., Ní Áinle, F., Rosenkranz, S., and Pruszczyk, P. (2021). Optimal follow-up after acute pulmonary embolism: A position paper of the European Society of Cardiology Working Group on Pulmonary Circulation and Right Ventricular Function, in collaboration with the European Society of Cardiology Working Group on Atherosclerosis and Vascular Biology, endorsed by the European Respiratory Society, *European Heart Journal*, 43(3), pp. 183–189.

Konstantinides, S.V., Barco, S., Rosenkranz, S., Lankeit, M., Held. M., Gerhardt, F., Bruch, L., Ewert, R., Faehling, M., Freise, J., Ghofrani, H.A., Grünig, E., Halank, M., Heydenreich, N., Hoeper, M.M., Leuchte, H.H., Mayer, E., Meyer, F.J., Neurohr, C., Opitz, C., Pinto, A., Seyfarth, H.J., Wachter, R., Zäpf, B., Wilkens, H., Binder, H., and Wild, P.S. (2016). Late outcomes after acute pulmonary embolism: Rationale and design of FOCUS, a prospective observational multicenter cohort study, *Journal of Thrombosis and Thrombolysis*, 42(4), pp. 600–609.

McCabe, C., Deboeck, G., Harvey, I., Ross, R.M., Gopalan, D., Screaton, N., and Pepke-Zaba, J. (2013). Inefficient exercise gas exchange identifies pulmonary hypertension in chronic thromboembolic obstruction following pulmonary embolism, *Thrombosis Research*, 132(6), pp. 659–665.

McCabe, C., Dimopoulos, K., Pitcher, A., Orchard, E., Price, L.C., Kempny, A., and Wort, S.J. (2020). Chronic thromboembolic disease following pulmonary embolism: Time for a fresh look at old clot, *European Respiratory Journal*, 55(4), pp. 3.

Zhuang, Y., Dai, L.F., and Chen, M.Q. (2021). Efficacy and safety of non-vitamin K antagonist oral anticoagulants for venous thromboembolism: A meta-analysis, *JRSM Open*, 12(6), pp. 1–14.

Chapter 15

Long-Term Breathlessness Despite Anticoagulation — What are the Treatment Options?

Wei Qi and David M. Systrom

Division of Pulmonary Critical Care Medicine, Brigham and Women's Hospital, Harvard Medical School, Boston, MA, USA

Abstract

Long-term breathlessness after acute pulmonary embolism (PE) is common and can negatively affect exercise capacity, functional status, and quality of life. Persistent dyspnoea after PE is collectively known as post-PE syndrome, manifesting clinically as chronic thromboembolic pulmonary hypertension (CTEPH), chronic thromboembolic disease (CTEPD), post-PE cardiac, and functional impairments. Pathophysiologic mechanisms underlying these clinical domains include abnormal ventilation–perfusion matching, increased physiologic deadspace fraction, abnormal pulmonary vascular response, and right ventricular uncoupling during exercise among others, which can be elucidated using invasive cardiopulmonary exercise testing. Pulmonary endarterectomy is the treatment of choice for CTEPH patients with operable disease, and balloon pulmonary angioplasty has been shown to improve haemodynamics and quality-of-life in non-operable patients. Medical therapy is indicated in patients with persistent or recurrent pulmonary hypertension (PH) after PEA and non-operable patients, with riociguat being the first approved therapy. Adjunctive therapies, especially cardio-pulmonary rehabilitation, have also shown benefit. In this complex and often under-recognised population of patients, a high index of suspicion for screening and diagnosis, a low threshold for referral to an expert centre, and a multidisciplinary approach to management are vital for providing optimal care.

Introduction

Long-term breathlessness after acute pulmonary embolism (PE) is common and encompasses a range of clinical domains and pathophysiologic mechanisms, making it difficult to detect, diagnose, and treat patients with debilitating and serious complications such as chronic thromboembolic pulmonary hypertension (CTEPH). Therefore, a high index of suspicion for screening and diagnosis, a low threshold for referral to an expert centre, and a multidisciplinary approach are needed to optimise care in this vulnerable population. This chapter aims to outline the clinical domains and pathophysiologic mechanisms that underlie long-term breathlessness in post-PE patients and to describe the interventional, medical, and rehabilitative approaches to management.

Post-PE Syndrome

Studies have shown that approximately 40–60% of acute PE survivors experience persistent dyspnoea and functional limitations, even with adequate therapeutic anticoagulation of at least 3 months. The symptoms of persistent or worsening dyspnoea, exertional intolerance, anxiety, depression, functional limitations, and decreased quality of life are collectively known as post-PE syndrome, which can be broadly categorised into the following clinical domains: CTEPH, chronic thromboembolic disease (CTEPD), post-PE cardiac impairment, and post-PE functional impairment (Table 1).

The incidence of CTEPH is estimated to be approximately 2–4% among acute PE survivors, with a prevalence of 8–40 cases per million. These are likely underestimations, however, due to paucity of early symptoms and difficulty differentiating symptoms of acute PE from development of long-term sequelae CTEPH is the most serious long-term complication after acute PE. It is characterised by fibrotic organisation of unresolved pulmonary thromboemboli leading to persistent obstruction of pulmonary arteries, progressive pulmonary arterial remodelling and vasculopathy, increased pulmonary vascular resistance, pulmonary hypertension (PH), and ultimately right ventricular dysfunction and failure. The condition is diagnosed in a dyspnoeic post-PE patient by fulfilling both imaging and haemodynamic criteria after 3 months of therapeutic anticoagulation. The imaging criteria are met by abnormal ventilation–perfusion scintigraphy, computed tomography or pulmonary angiography, and the haemodynamic criteria are fulfilled by a mean pulmonary arterial pressure (mPAP) ≥25 mmHg and a pulmonary capillary wedge pressure ≤15 mmHg on resting right heart catheterisation. Whether the newly proposed PH definition with an mPAP cut-off value of 20 mmHg should be applied to the diagnosis of CTEPH is still under consideration. The etiology of persistent dyspnoea after acute PE can be difficult to elucidate when resting right heart catheterisation reveals normal haemodynamics, however, and cardiopulmonary exercise testing (CPET) can help differentiate the potential mechanisms of unexplained dyspnoea. CTEPD, for instance, is a condition disparate from CTEPH in which dyspnoeic post-PE patients are found to have persistent perfusion defects without PH at rest but exhibit abnormal pulmonary vascular and gas exchange responses on CPET.

In addition to CTEPH and CTEPD, post-PE cardiac and functional impairments are common and may coexist with the other clinical domains. Right ventricular (RV) dysfunction is postulated to result from an inflammatory response to acute PE, triggered by a combination of factors including RV myocyte stretch, shear forces, impaired perfusion, increased metabolic demand, and resultant myocardial fibrosis. On echocardiography, RV dysfunction may manifest as RV hypokinesis or dilation. Left ventricular (LV) dysfunction has also been found among PE survivors, with left-sided diastolic dysfunction being the most prevalent echocardiographic abnormality. Additionally, biventricular function has been shown to be impaired during exercise, resulting in exertional intolerance.

Post-PE functional impairment encompasses new or worsening dyspnoea, exertional intolerance, functional limitations after acute PE, as well as venous thromboembolism (VTE)-related mental health problems such as anxiety, depression, and post-thrombotic panic syndrome. The ELOPE study, a multicentre, prospective cohort study evaluating exercise limitation, health-related quality of life, and dyspnoea after acute PE found that half of post-PE patients had exercise limitation at 1 year, defined by percent-predicted peak oxygen uptake (VO_2) <80% on CPET, which was associated with poorer quality of life, higher dyspnoea scores, and worse 6-minute walk distance (6MWD). Muscle deconditioning was felt to be a major contributor to exercise limitation. Lastly, untreated anxiety and depression can lead to less physical activity and further worsening of a deconditioned state.

Physiological Mechanisms

Exertional capacity is often impaired by several physiologic defects in post-PE patients, with significant heterogeneity between patients. Multiple studies have suggested that the traditional metrics of cardiopulmonary exercise testing, namely ventilatory and circulatory limitations, might not sufficiently explain the physiologic deficits that underlie post-PE dyspnoea, and that peak VO_2 is not a sensitive physiologic marker of dyspnoea after PE. Instead, the following mechanisms, including ventilation–perfusion mismatch, right ventricular dysfunction and uncoupling, chronotropic incompetence, and impaired peripheral extraction, are associated with exertional capacity in studies involving exercise testing and dyspneic post-PE subjects (Table 1).

Ventilation–perfusion (V/Q) mismatch

A rise in ventilation during exercise is determined by variables related to cellular metabolism, including decreased arterial O_2 content, lactic acidemia, and increased mixed-venous CO_2 load. Minute ventilation (V_E) with respect to CO_2 production (VCO_2) represents ventilatory efficiency. Ventilatory inefficiency, as reflected by a higher V_E/VCO_2

Table 1. Clinical domains and physiological mechanisms of post-PE syndrome.

Post-PE syndrome	
Clinical domains	Physiological mechanisms
• CTEPH	• V/Q mismatch
• CTEPD	• RV dysfunction and uncoupling
• Post-PE cardiac impairment	• Chronotropic incompetence
• Post-PE functional impairment	• Impaired peripheral extraction

slope, or a higher V_E/VCO_2 ratio at the anaerobic threshold (AT), is a hallmark of many cardiopulmonary diseases, indicating increased ventilation for a given CO_2 output. Lower ventilatory efficiency is found in patients with CTEPH both at rest and at peak exercise, and in some studies both V_E/VCO_2 slope and V_E/VCO_2 ratio at AT were significantly higher than other forms of PH such as pulmonary arterial hypertension (PAH).

From rest to maximal exercise, physiologic dead-space fraction (V_D/V_T) progressively decreases, with a normal response being $V_D/V_T < 20\%$ at peak exercise. The steady increase in tidal volume with increasing work rate, and decreased alveolar dead space accompanied by only minimal increases in anatomic dead-space, explains the normal drop in V_D/V_T with exercise. Ventilatory inefficiency in CTEPH patients is thought to be attributable to exercise hyperventilation and increased V_D/V_T, the latter explained by a failure of adequate recruitment of the pulmonary capillary bed on exercise due to persistent vascular obstruction and a shift towards higher ventilation–perfusion ratios. Dead-space fraction is suggested by multiple studies to contribute more towards ventilatory inefficiency in CTEPH than other forms of PH. Additionally, it predicts a diagnosis of CTEPH with high sensitivity and specificity and correlated well with severity of haemodynamic derangement. Larger dead-space fraction has also been shown to be associated with decreased exercise capacity, worse NYHA functional class, and increased mortality in patients with CTEPH. In addition to increased dead-space fraction, hyperventilation from RV outflow stretch-receptor activation, dynamic arterial O_2 desaturation, and exercise lactic acidemia have been postulated to contribute to ventilatory inefficiency.

Ventilation–perfusion mismatch also negatively impacts gas exchange, as demonstrated by lower arterial partial pressure of oxygen (P_aO_2) and higher alveolar-arterial (A-a) gradients in CTEPH patients compared with PAH patients, especially during exercise. One theory to explain such an observed difference is that the non-uniform vascular obstruction in CTEPH results in more pronounced blood flow redistribution and dead-space effect, while more uniformly distributed microvascular disease in PAH minimises this effect. Similarly, patients with CTEPD also exhibit abnormal ventilatory efficiency, elevated dead-space fraction, and impaired gas exchange compared to healthy subjects, but not as severe as CTEPH patients, representing an intermediary pathophenotype.

RV dysfunction and uncoupling

The right ventricle and its interaction with the pulmonary circulation are important determinants of exertional capacity. In post-PE patients with persistent dyspnoea, both RV function and coupling with the pulmonary vasculature are impaired. While impaired RV function can be readily detected in patients with CTEPH by resting imaging and haemodynamic evaluations, RV chamber morphology and contractility may be preserved in CTEPD patients at rest. Therefore, exercise testing may be required for the assessment of possible RV dysfunction and uncoupling in patients with post-PE dyspnoea.

During upright exercise in healthy individuals, cardiac output increases through increased heart rate and stroke volume. Stroke volume is augmented by increased venous return from contracting muscles as well as increased cardiac contractility. End-systolic volume (ESV) is decreased, reflecting a healthy contractile reserve, and end-diastolic volume (EDV) is unchanged or slightly decreased at peak exercise due to reduced filling times. Additionally, during early exercise, the pulmonary vasculature dilates, and the recruitment of previously under-perfused pulmonary vascular beds occurs in conjunction with increased RV cardiac output, thereby decreasing pulmonary vascular resistance (PVR) and increasing pulmonary arterial compliance. RV afterload is determined by the dynamic interplay between pulmonary arterial compliance, PVR, and wave reflection. Pulmonary arterial compliance, or the distensibility of the pulmonary vasculature in response to increases in pressure, is inversely related to PVR. While PVR represents mean pressure divided by mean flow, pulmonary arterial compliance better incorporates the pulsatile nature of the pulmonary circulation. Slight increases in PVR can result in large reductions in compliance, making pulmonary arterial compliance a more meaningful predictor of abnormal pulmonary vascular response to exercise.

Persistent vascular obstruction from organised fibrotic thrombi in post-PE patients can decrease pulmonary arterial compliance and increase both resistive and pulsatile RV afterload. This can in turn negatively affect adaptive cardiac output augmentation during exercise by elevating RV end-diastolic and ESVs as well as impairing RV contractility. The reduced RV contractile reserve in the presence of an increased RV afterload represents a process of uncoupling between the RV and pulmonary circulation, which eventually leads to impaired oxygen delivery and exertional intolerance.

Chronotropic incompetence and impaired peripheral extraction

Chronotropic incompetence is another mechanism that has been shown to impede cardiac output augmentation during exercise. Down-regulation of β-adrenergic receptors in the right ventricle has been shown to occur in PAH in proportion to severity of disease. It has also been postulated that chronic RV pressure overload causing right atrial stretch may eventually lead to remodelling of the right atrium and sinus node. These putative pathophysiologic mechanisms are often compounded by the use of negative chronotropic medications, leading to chronotropic incompetence and exertional intolerance in post-PE patients.

Normal functional capacity requires adequate interaction between central and peripheral mechanisms to ensure O_2 delivery and O_2 extraction, and perturbations in these processes may result in exertional intolerance and functional limitations. In addition to central processes affecting O_2 delivery, exercise testing in CTEPH patients also found that O_2 extraction in the periphery may be negatively impacted, evidenced by reduced skeletal muscle diffusion capacity. This impairment persists despite improvements in haemodynamics and RV function in patients who received surgical or percutaneous intervention for CTEPH, suggesting that physical deconditioning due to inactivity and other causes, such as major surgery and an inflammatory milieu, may contribute to impaired peripheral extraction.

Management

Pulmonary endarterectomy

CTEPH is potentially curable by pulmonary endarterectomy (PEA). Operable CTEPH is often characterised by surgically accessible, proximal forms of disease involving large elastic vessels down to the segmental artery level, with high disease burden and no major contraindication to surgery. As operability is a key decision in assessing treatment options in CTEPH patients, it should be determined by a multidisciplinary team including PH specialists, radiologists, surgeons, and interventionalists (Figure 1).

Pulmonary endarterectomy is the guideline-recommended treatment of choice for patients with CTEPH, one with the most published evidence. It is a major surgical procedure requiring general anaesthesia, median

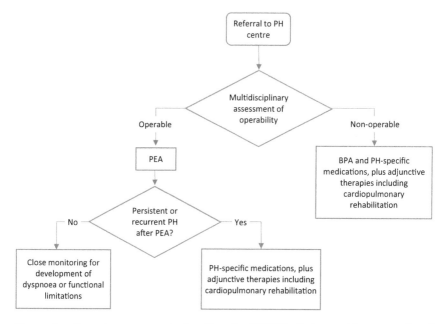

Figure 1.   General management algorithm for CTEPH. Patients with suspected and confirmed CTEPH should undergo referral to a PH centre for multidisciplinary evaluation of operability. Pulmonary endarterectomy is the treatment of choice for operable CTEPH. If persistent or recurrent PH occurs post-PEA, PH-specific medications should be considered, as well as adjunctive therapies including cardiopulmonary rehabilitation. Non-operable CTEPH patients should be evaluated for BPA, PH-specific medications, and should be offered appropriate adjunctive therapies including cardiopulmonary rehabilitation.

sternotomy, deep hypothermic circulatory arrest, and cardiopulmonary bypass. Unlike surgical embolectomy for acute PE, PEA requires a bloodless field achieved by deep hypothermic circulatory arrest, during which surgeons perform complete endarterectomy through the medial layer of pulmonary arteries with the goal to clear all obstructive material. Since the original technique was popularised by the team from University of California at San Diego, experienced surgeons now can not only remove proximal laminated thrombi, but are also able reach the subsegmental level and remove distal webs and occlusions in vessels as small as 1–2 mm. Post-operatively, patients require intensive care with mechanical ventilation, inotropic support and aggressive diuresis, followed by at least one week of hospitalisation, with full recovery usually taking 2–3 months.

Pulmonary endarterectomy has the most evidence for efficacy for improvements in both haemodynamics and functional status, with discernable improvements occurring almost immediately following surgery. The largest single centre retrospective cohort of patients who underwent PEA found an mPAP decline from 45.5 mmHg before surgery to 26.0 mmHg after, with PVR decreasing from 719.0 to 253.4 dynes/s/cm⁵. Six-Minute Walk Distance (in, meters) was also found to increase from 362 to 459 m in an international CTEPH registry of 386 patients undergoing PEA. In a long-term follow up of 880 patients following PEA, World Health Organization (WHO) Functional Class (1/2/3/4, %) were improved from 0/9/68/23 to 34/47/15/0. In CTEPD patients, PEA similarly resulted in significant improvement in symptoms and quality of life.

In the original international CTEPH registry including 386 patients who underwent PEA at 17 centres from 2007 to 2009, in-hospital mortality was 4.7%. A single specialist centre found in-hospital mortality to be even lower at 2.2% for 500 patients who underwent PEA. While in-hospital mortality is relatively low, perioperative complications have been recorded in up to half of patients in some studies. Specific complications pertaining to PEA include right ventricular failure, reperfusion lung injury, airway haemorrhage and residual PH, and in severe cases may require veno-venous (VV-) or veno-arterial (VA-) extracorporeal membrane oxygenation (ECMO) as bridge to recovery, or in select candidates with severe persistent PH, bridge to emergency lung transplantation. While patients undergoing PEA at high-volume centres have excellent long-term survival of around 70% at 10 years as shown in longitudinal studies, residual PH was common. Approximately half of patients have an mPAP greater than 25 mmHg at 6 months following PEA surgery. Thus, post-PEA patients require careful follow up and some may require additional therapy even after surgery.

Balloon pulmonary angioplasty

Although PEA is the treatment of choice and potentially curative for CTEPH, about one-third of patients have non-operable disease, and intervention with balloon pulmonary angioplasty (BPA) should be considered. Non-operable CTEPH involves distal lesions that reside predominantly beyond the segmental level, presents in a distribution that is surgically inaccessible, or harbours a disease burden that fails to justify operative risks. BPA was first described in 2001 by Feinstein and Landzberg in a series of 18 patients with non-operable CTEPH who underwent balloon dilatation of the pulmonary arteries. Due to high rate of short-term mortality (30-day, 5.5%) and frequency of major complications, with 11 patients developing reperfusion pulmonary edema and 3 patients requiring mechanical ventilation, the technique was initially abandoned. However, over the course of the following decade, BPA technique was refined by interventionalists in Japan and Europe by careful selection of balloon size, titration of number of treated lesions to the level of mPAP, which resulted in improved outcomes for patients with non-operable CTEPH and a resurgence for its use. In the 2015 European Society of Cardiology (ESC) and the European Respiratory Society (ERS) Guidelines for diagnosis and treatment of PH, BPA was included as a class IIb recommendation for patients with CTEPH who have inaccessible disease or prohibitive risk for PEA surgery.

In the modern BPA technique, jugular or femoral venous sheaths are inserted under local anaesthesia, and balloon-mounted catheters are introduced over a guidewire into the diseased pulmonary segmental and subsegmental arteries. The balloon is then serially inflated in vessels to expand stenotic or obstructive lesions and improve distal pulmonary blood flow. A complete treatment course requires 4–6 BPA sessions in order to sufficiently reduce pulmonary vascular resistance, decrease right ventricular afterload, and improve right ventricular function.

Meta-analysis of observational studies suggests that BPA may have similar efficacy to PEA and is superior to medical therapy alone in CTEPH patients. Haemodynamic and symptomatic improvements post-BPA are significant but not immediate, due to time required for vascular healing and favourable vessel remodelling beyond simple opening of obstructed vessels. Systematic reviews found that BPA treatments delivered through on average 2.5–6.6 sessions, mPAP reduced by 14.2 mmHg and PVR declined by 303.5 dynes/s/cm^5. Six-minute walk distance, similarly, was found to be increased by 67.3 m. A minimal important difference (MID) in 6MWD associated with an impact on quality-of-life measures was estimated to be 33 m in PAH patients. While the MID of 33 m might not be necessarily applicable to CTEPH patients, a 6MWD improvement doubled that of MID is suggestive of a substantial improvement in quality of life post-BPA. BPA effects have been shown to be durable at 5 years, with only rare incidences of restenosis.

Percutaneous BPA, though invasive, is a safe procedure with reported short- and long-term mortality being 1.9% and 5.7%, respectively. Complications can occur at a higher rate in approximately 10% of procedures, often due to lung reperfusion injury, haemoptysis, with severe cases requiring non-invasive ventilation, endotracheal intubation, or mechanical circulatory support. If haemoptysis is due to distal wire exit, prolonged balloon inflation, reversal of anticoagulation, and occasionally transcatheter gel or coil embolisation may be required. Percutaneous BPA has been demonstrated to be safe and effective in CTEPD as well, with low rates of complications and improvements in haemodynamic measurements as well as functional status.

Medical therapy

In addition to percutaneous BPA, medical therapy with PH-targeted medications is often employed for the treatment of non-operable CTEPH. In fact, medical therapy is thought to be complementary to BPA by addressing distal microvasculopathy, while BPA relieves segmental and subsegmental disease. Additionally, patients with persistent or recurrent PH after PEA may be candidates for PH-targeted therapy.

Riociguat, an enteral soluble guanylate cyclase stimulator, has been shown to improve haemodynamics and exertional capacity. Riociguat acts by both independently stimulating soluble guanylate cyclase and augmenting the sensitivity of guanylate cyclase to nitric oxide, thereby increasing the levels of cyclic guanosine monophosphate which then mediates vasodilatory, antiproliferative, and antifibrotic downstream effects. In a randomised, double-blind, placebo-controlled study of patients with non-operable CTEPH or persistent or recurrent PH after PEA, treatment with riociguat after 16 weeks led to a decrease in PVR of 226 dynes/s/cm^5, a mean increase in 6MWD of 39 m, and was also associated with improvements in NT-ProBNP and WHO Functional Class. The Food and Drug Administration (FDA), as well as the European Medicines Agency, approved riociguat for the treatment of adults with persistent or recurrent CTEPH after surgical treatment or non-operable CTEPH.

Additionally, macitentan, an endothelin receptor antagonist, was shown to significantly improve PVR in patients with non-operable CTEPH and was well tolerated. More recently, a multicentres, randomised, double-blind controlled trial demonstrated that treatment with subcutaneous

Treprostinil was safe and improved exercise capacity in patients with non-operable CTEPH or persistent or recurrent PH after PEA. Subcutaneous Treprostinil, a prostacyclin analogue, is a parenteral alternative for patients who cannot tolerate other therapies or need combination treatment. The concept of using PH-targeted therapy as a bridge to intervention remains an area of uncertainty to date, as evidence of safety and efficacy is currently lacking.

In addition to PH-targeted therapies, optimal medical treatment for CTEPH also involves lifelong anticoagulation, diuretics, and supplemental oxygen in cases of hypoxemia. Adjunctive therapies including cardiopulmonary rehabilitation are also important especially in patients with persistent dyspnoea despite improvement in haemodynamics post-intervention. Cardiac rehabilitation improved peak VO_2 in patients with non-operable CTEPH who underwent BPA intervention, and health-related quality of life showed a trend towards improvement in this group as well. Additionally, combined cycling and resistance training has been shown to improve muscle strength, increase number of capillaries and oxidative activity in skeletal muscles of patients with PAH. Therefore, cardiopulmonary rehabilitation should be offered to patients with post-PE dyspnoea, especially in those with deconditioning. Lastly, VTE-related mental health issues, such as post-thrombotic panic syndrome and anxiety, can exacerbate dyspnoea, deconditioning, and significantly limit quality of life. Therefore, early referral for evaluation and treatment for these psychiatric comorbidities should be considered.

Conclusion

Long-term breathlessness after acute PE is also known as post-PE syndrome, encompassing CTEPH, CTEPD, post-PE cardiac, and functional impairments. Post-PE syndrome is common and can severely limit exercise capacity, functional status, and quality of life. Diagnosing post-PE syndrome requires a multimodal approach, involving imaging, haemodynamic, functional, and mental health screening modalities. Patients with suspicion for CTEPH and CTEPD should undergo early referral to PH centres for multidisciplinary evaluation and treatment planning. Exercise testing can help detect abnormal V/Q matching, abnormal pulmonary vascular response, and RV uncoupling during exercise, especially in dyspneic patients with normal resting haemodynamics. Pulmonary endarterectomy is the treatment of choice for CTEPH patients with operable disease. In patients with non-operable disease, BPA has been shown to improve haemodynamics and quality-of-life. Medical therapy is indicated in patients with persistent or recurrent PH after PEA and non-operable patients, with riociguat being the FDA-approved therapy. Adjunctive therapies, especially cardiopulmonary rehabilitation, have also shown benefit. Post-PE syndrome is a debilitating and serious group of conditions and remains an area of active and ongoing research. With increasing awareness, a multidisciplinary approach, and advancements in interventional and medical therapies, patient outcomes continue to improve.

Bibliography

Cannon, J.E., Su, L., Kiely, D.G. *et al.* (2016). Dynamic risk stratification of patient long-term outcome after pulmonary endarterectomy: Results From the United Kingdom National Cohort, *Circulation*, 133(18), pp. 1761–1771.

Feinstein, J.A., Goldhaber, S.Z., Lock, J.E., Fernandes, S.M., and Landzberg, M.J. (2001). Balloon pulmonary angioplasty for treatment of chronic thromboembolic pulmonary hypertension, *Circulation*, 103(1), pp. 10–13.

Ghofrani, H.A., D'Armini, A.M., Grimminger, F. *et al.* (2013). Riociguat for the treatment of chronic thromboembolic pulmonary hypertension, The *New England Journal of Medicine*, 369(4), pp. 319–329.

Ghofrani, H.A., Simonneau, G., D'Armini, A.M. *et al.* (2017). Macitentan for the treatment of inoperable chronic thromboembolic pulmonary hypertension (MERIT-1): Results from the multicentre, phase 2, randomised, double-blind, placebo-controlled study, *The Lancet Respiratory Medicine*, 5(10), pp. 785–794.

Kahn, S.R., Hirsch, A.M., Akaberi, A. *et al.* (2017). Functional and exercise limitations after a first episode of pulmonary embolism: Results of the ELOPE prospective cohort study, *Chest*, 151(5), pp. 1058–1068.

Khan, M.S., Amin, E., Memon, M.M. *et al.* (2019). Meta-analysis of use of balloon pulmonary angioplasty in patients with inoperable chronic thromboembolic pulmonary hypertension, *International Journal of Cardiology*, 291, pp. 134–139.

Madani, M.M., Auger, W.R., Pretorius, V. *et al.* (2012). Pulmonary endarterectomy: Recent changes in a single institution's experience of more than 2,700 patients, *The Annals of Thoracic Surgery*, 94(1), pp. 97–103.

Mathai, S.C., Puhan, M.A., Lam, D., and Wise, R.A. (2012). The minimal important difference in the 6-minute walk test for patients with pulmonary arterial hypertension, *American Journal of Respiratory and Critical Care Medicine*, 186(5), pp. 428–433.

Mayer, E., Jenkins, D., Lindner, J. *et al.* (2011). Surgical management and outcome of patients with chronic thromboembolic pulmonary hypertension: Results from an international prospective registry, *The Journal Thoracic Cardiovascular Surgery*, 141(3), pp. 702–710.

Sadushi-Kolici, R., Jansa, P., Kopec, G. *et al.* (2019). Subcutaneous treprostinil for the treatment of severe non-operable chronic thromboembolic pulmonary hypertension (CTREPH): A double-blind, phase 3, randomised controlled trial, *The Lancet Respiratory Medicine*, 7(3), pp. 239–248.

Chapter 16

COVID-19-Associated Thrombosis

Christina Crossette-Thambiah*, **Laura C. Price**†,
and Deepa J. Arachchillage*

Imperial College Healthcare NHS Trust, London, UK

†*Department of Cardiology, Royal Brompton and Harefield Hospitals,
Guy's and St Thomas' NHS Foundation Trust, London, UK*

Abstract

COVID-19 caused by the severe acute respiratory syndrome coronavirus 2 (SARS-CoV-2) is a global pandemic. The clinical presentations of COVID-19 are highly variable, ranging from asymptomatic to severe respiratory failure, with or without multiorgan failure leading to death. Interactions between the innate immune system, coagulation activation, and endothelial dysfunction in individuals with COVID-19 together create a highly hypercoagulable environment that we are still attempting to fully discern. This highly prothrombotic drive manifests as venous thromboembolism affecting the pulmonary vasculature both with *in situ* thrombosis and pulmonary embolism and deep vein thrombosis as well as arterial thrombosis such as stroke and myocardial infarction. In this chapter, we aim to provide the overview of the pathophysiology of thrombosis, investigations and strategies of prevention and management and follow-up mainly of venous thromboembolism in patients requiring hospitalisation due to COVID-19.

Introduction

Coagulation dysfunction and thrombosis are major complications in patients with COVID-19 and associated with poor prognosis. Coagulation abnormalities are a well-known feature of severe infections but virtually in all reports both these changes and thrombosis, despite standard thromboprophylaxis, are more common in COVID-19 than in other pneumonias. In a meta-analysis of 7 studies, including 1,783 patients with adult respiratory distress syndrome (ARDS) from causes other than COVID-19, the incidence of venous thromboembolism (VTE) was 12.7%. Thrombotic complications are much higher in critically ill patients treated in intensive care units (ICU) compared to those managed in the wards or the community (28% thrombotic events in patients treated in ICU compared to 7% in ward-treated patients). Understanding and managing thrombosis in COVID-19 therefore remains of utmost importance.

Interactions between the innate immune system, coagulation activation and endothelial dysfunction in individuals with COVID-19 together create a highly hypercoagulable environment that we are still attempting to fully discern. This highly prothrombotic drive manifests as VTE affecting the pulmonary vasculature both with *in situ* thrombosis and pulmonary embolism and deep vein thrombosis (DVT) as well as arterial thrombosis such as stroke and myocardial infarction. In this chapter, we aim to provide the overview of the pathophysiology of thrombosis, investigations and strategies of prevention and management mainly of VTE in patients requiring hospitalisation due to COVID-19.

Pathogenesis

SARS-CoV-2 is a zoonotic virus capable of transmission from human to human via transfer through aerosols or contaminated surfaces. The role of angiotensin-converting enzyme 2 (ACE2) receptor has been central to the primary mechanism proposed in SARS-CoV-2 pathogenesis. The ACE2 receptor is differentially expressed on various tissues, including respiratory tract cells, gastrointestinal tract cells and endothelial cells among others. ACE2 acts as a membrane receptor when the viral spike protein binds to it and successful viral entry into the cells requires transmembrane serine protease 2 (TMPRSS2) which cleaves and activates ACE2. Recently, it has been demonstrated that TMPRSS2 is expressed in the endothelial cells lining the lungs which may well support the predominance of pulmonary complications in COVID-19. Furthermore, TMPRSS2 expression was increased in the bronchial epithelial cells of male patients compared with female patients, a possible explanation for the increased risk in males for severe disease and thrombotic complications. Notably, SARS-CoV-2 infection results in death and internalisation of ACE2 receptors causing reduced ACE2 activity and given its role in the renin angiotensin aldosterone system a reduction in ACE2 will ultimately upregulate angiotensin II activity. Angiotensin II has procoagulant activity via stimulation of the tissue factor (TF) pathway, increasing tissue plasminogen activator inhibitor type 1 (PAI-1) activity, and inhibiting tissue plasminogen activator (tPA) expression. Here we will discuss this and other plausible pathogenic mechanisms at play in COVID-19-associated thrombosis.

Vascular endothelial injury

Virus-induced endothelial damage and inflammation may well be a central explanation of the pathogenesis of thrombotic complications of COVID-19. It has been demonstrated that pulmonary vascular endothelialitis, thrombosis, and intussusceptive angiogenesis occurs more intensely in patients infected with SARS-CoV-2 than other viral infections or interstitial pneumonias.

Inflammation is a well-established driver of coagulation activation leading to thrombosis via multiple mechanisms. Firstly, systemic inflammatory mediators drive production of coagulation factors from the liver and from endothelium creating a procoagulant state. They also upregulate TF expression on leucocytes and endothelial cells triggering the coagulation cascade. Secondly, endothelial activation results in down regulation of surface anticoagulant molecules such as thrombomodulin and TFPI potentiating the procoagulant effects and allowing high levels of thrombin generation. In the lungs, endothelial activation may be further stimulated by hypoxia. Thirdly, endothelial activation releases ultra large multimers of von Willebrand factor (VWF) and upregulation of adhesion molecules resulting in platelet capture, localising thrombin formation to the vessel wall, and formation of thrombus. Finally, activation of neutrophils causes them to unravel and extrude their DNA in neutrophil extracellular traps (NETs). These activate platelets, bind VWF, and provide a negatively charged surface for the contact activation system to further drive thrombin generation.

Thrombi can therefore be a complex mixture of VWF, platelets, fibrin, and DNA perhaps requiring an equally complex approach to therapy.

Immunothrombosis

Thrombosis as a component of the innate immune response against pathogens is called immunothrombosis which can lead to fatal complications. Thrombo-inflammation is driven by the interactions between macrophages, polymorphonuclear cells, platelets, coagulation factors, and immunoeffector proteins resulting in systemic hypercoagulation. Physiologically this is a complementary, balanced interplay but becomes dysregulated and leads to excess thrombus formation in severe infection including SARS-CoV-2. When cells are infected with SARS-CoV-2 they release pathogen-associated molecular pattern (PAMPs), and damage-associated molecular patterns (DAMPs) which cause inflammation. An immune response is triggered, and pro-inflammatory cytokines are released. Patients with SARS-CoV-2 have raised levels of IL-6, IL-2, and interferon-gamma which can enhance TF expression. IL-6 and IFN-γ specifically has been shown to increase platelet production in SARS-COV-2 infected patients while IL-2 can impact fibrinolysis as discussed later.

The activation of multiple cellular and humoral inflammatory system amplification pathways in turn activate various coagulation pathways such as contact factor activations, fibrinolytic pathway activation, and complement activation. Aside from these pathways, polymorphonuclear and mononuclear-driven prothrombotic pathways also play a role. For example, polymorphonuclear cells cam stimulate formation of NETs, which can stimulate coagulation activation via factor XII and via inhibition of anticoagulant proteins. This has been demonstrated in COVID-19 patients where formation of NETs was associated with increased thrombotic complications.

Fibrin deposition and fibrinolysis

Along with fibrin formation in thrombi, ARDS, a central complication in patients with COVID-19, is characterised by increased alveolar capillary permeability and exudation of fluid rich in inflammatory cells, pro-inflammatory cytokines such as IL-6 and TNF-α, and coagulation factors including fibrinogen. This leads to fibrin deposition in the air spaces and lung parenchyma which is observed in patients with COVID-19. Fibrin formation will itself trigger activation of fibrinolysis, by binding tPA and plasminogen to generate plasmin but uPA-uPAR which are predominantly extravascular and are known to be active on lung epithelia may also contribute. Fibrinolytic activation is regulated by plasminogen activator inhibitor 1 (PAI-1), the principal inhibitor of tissue-type plasminogen activator (tPA) and urokinase-type plasminogen activator (uPA) which is expressed by endothelial cells, epithelial cells, monocytes, and macrophages. Endothelial and platelet activation releases PAI-1 and down regulates fibrinolysis. Interestingly, Angiotensin II is reported to upregulate PAI-1 expression in EC. The functional capacity of the fibrinolytic system is an important determinant of fibrin deposition.

Assessment of fibrinolysis using thromboelastography (TEG 6, Haemonetics®, UK) in patients with severe COVID-19, have shown absent fibrinolysis at 30 minutes to be a universal finding (Figure 1). This phenomenon, described as "fibrinolysis shutdown", has been shown to be a predictor of first and recurrent PE, micro and macrovascular thrombosis and potentially alveolar fibrin deposition. High expression of PAI-1 may cause longer-term problems as it facilitates tissue fibrosis by inhibiting plasmin mediated activation of tissue matrix metalloproteases.

Platelets

Thrombocytopenia is present in less than a fifth of COVID-19 patients compared to over half of patients presenting with non-COVID-19 ARDS. However, platelet activation may play an important part in the thrombotic component of COVID-19 and may arise via a number of mechanisms. Firstly, release of ultra large VWF multimers from activated EC may capture platelets on the endothelial surface. Secondly, systemic platelet activation may occur via IL-6 or by direct interaction with viruses via platelet Toll-like receptor recognition of pathogen or damage-associated molecular patterns (PAMPs and DAMPs).

In keeping with this hypothesis, our assessment of platelet function using the Multiplate analyser (Roche Diagnostics, UK), found hyperactive platelets to be a major feature of mechanically ventilated patients admitted to intensive with COVID-19 pneumonia (Figure 2).

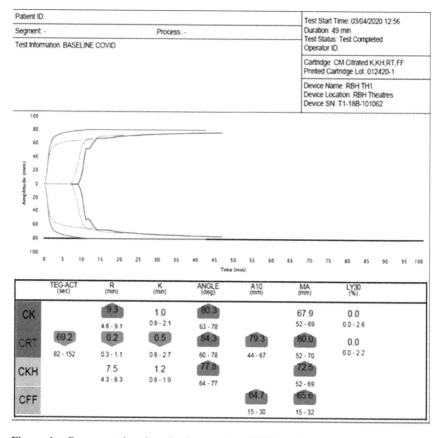

Figure 1. Representative thromboelastography (TEG) tracings of a ventilated patient with coronavirus disease (COVID-19) The patient TEG shows universal hypercoagulability, with higher a-angle and maximal amplitude (MA), and absent fibrinolysis at 30 minutes (LY30 = 0%). The most frequently used parameters in TEG include reaction time, which reflects the time of latency from the start of the test to initial fibrin formation, which is prolonged if the patient is on an anticoagulant or has a coagulation factor deficiency. Heparinase TEG (CKH) eliminates the effect of heparin. The alpha-angle measures the speed at which fibrin buildup and cross-linking takes place and hence assesses the rate of clot formation but also provides information on fibrin formation and cross-linking. The MA is a measure of the ultimate strength of the fibrin clot, that is, the overall stability of the clot. This is dependent on platelets (80%) and fibrin (20%) interactions.

Notes: A10: amplitude 10 minutes after the time blood starts to clot; ACT: activated clotting time; CFF: citrated blood sample activated by the functional fibrinogen test; CK: citrated blood sample activated with kaolin; CKH: citrated blood sample activated with kaolin and heparinase; CRT: citrated blood sample activated with RapidTEG; K: coagulation time (min); LY30: percentage lysis at 30 minutes after MA; R: reaction time.

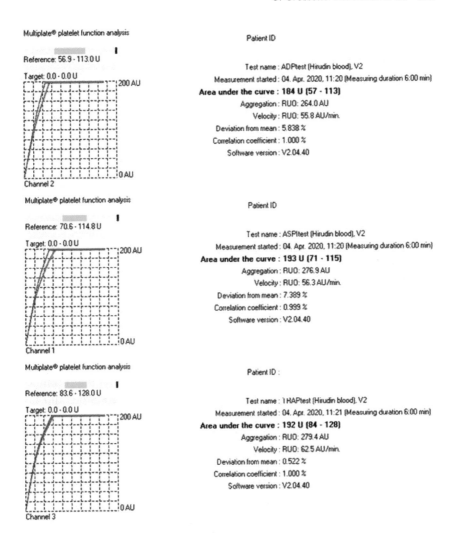

Figure 2. Platelet multiplate showing super active platelets across all three channels (ASPI test, ADP test and TRAP test) in a patient with severe COVID-19. Red and blue lines in each graph indicate the two pairs of sensor electrodes, each of which measures change in impedance based on aggregation of platelets in channel. Duplicate sensors serve as an integrated quality control and the difference of each curve is also calculated, and a difference of less than 20% is accepted which was the case in all tested patients. All three channels showed hyperaggregation of platelets demonstrating platelet activation.

Complement

The complement system has also been implicated in COVID-19 thrombosis and is a part of the immune response to SARS-CoV-2 infection. Continuous activation of the alternative and lectin pathways was noted in critically unwell COVID-19 patients with C5b-9 and C4d terminal fraction deposits found in the lung microvasculature and associated with microthrombosis. Furthermore, the membrane attack complex can trigger platelet activation and VWF release while C5a specifically can further stimulate prothrombotic drive by bringing about TF and PAI-1 production.

Autoantibodies including antiphospholipid antibodies

aPLs have been frequently detected in patients with COVID-19. In a meta-analysis and a systematic review to examine the prevalence of aPL and its clinical impact in patients with COVID-19 which included 21 studies with a total of 1159 patients, it was found that nearly half of patients with COVID-19 had aPL. The prevalence of aPL was even higher in patients with severe disease. However, this study did not detect any association between aPL positivity and disease outcomes including thrombosis, invasive ventilation or mortality. Additionally, these studies did not assess whether these antibodies are persistently positive after 12 weeks from the detection of acute infection. As transiently positive aPL is a well-known phenomenon in patients with acute infection, the significance of these antibodies in patients remains to be determined although some studies demonstrated aPL isolated from patients with COVID-19 causing thrombosis in a mouse model. However, further studies are required to identify the clinical and pathological role of aPL in COVID-19.

COVID-19: Thrombotic and thromboembolic clinical manifestations

The prevalence of VTE, including DVT and pulmonary embolism (PE), varies according to the severity of COVID-19 and is common in critically ill patients (Figure 3). An accurate prevalence of VTE associated with COVID-19 is unknown given that most studies did not include systematic

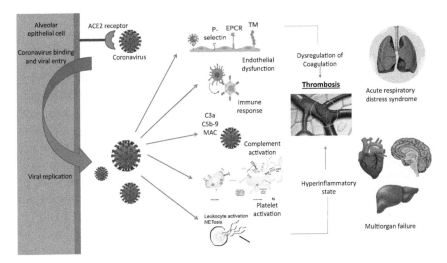

Figure 3. Mechanisms giving rise to thrombosis and multiorgan dysfunction in COVID-19. Binding of SARS-CoV-2 via the ACE2 receptor induces endothelial dysfunction and promotes the endothelial expression of proteins such as P-selectin, TF and VWF contributing to a hypercoagulable state. Binding of SARS-CoV-2 also results in mass innate immune cell infiltration and subsequent cytokine release, from these immune cells which can lead to induce the release of platelet contents, their activation and aggregation. Complement activation is another important inducer of coagulation with the Membrane attack complex (MAC) initiating cell lysis leading to microthrombi and coagulopathy. The neutrophil extracellular trap (NET)osis process can also stimulate thrombin production and fibrin deposition. Additionally, stimulation of autoantibody production including antiphospholipid antibodies may contribute to thrombosis. Overall, these mechanisms may act synergistically to create a hyperinflammatory state and dysregulation of coagulation which leads to thrombus formation, multiorgan failure, and eventually death.

and comprehensive investigation protocols. In a nationwide multicentre observational study in UK, which included 5,883 patients (≥18 years) admitted to 26 UK hospitals between 1 April 2020 and 31 July 2020, incidences of thrombosis (venous and arterial) and major bleeding (MB) were 5.4%, and 1.7%, respectively. The rates of VTE in patients treated on the ward and ICU were 119/5044 (2.4%) and 122/789 (15.5%), respectively. Arterial thrombosis rates in patients treated on the ward and ICU were 57/5044 (1.1%) and 22/789 (2.8%).

VTE: Screening and Diagnosis

Imaging

In terms of detecting venous thrombosis in patients with COVID-19, every effort should be made to assess the presence of a thrombosis objectively. However, this may be challenging in unstable patients with COVID-19 treated in the ICU. There is currently insufficient data in favour or against routine DVT screening using Doppler ultrasound (US) in patients with COVID-19, regardless of coagulation marker status. The benefits of routine screening may be early diagnosis of DVT and PE prevention. However, many of the patients diagnosed with PE do not have DVT in patients with COVID-19. The onset of PE is likely to follow both thromboembolic events from DVT as well as relate to local immunothrombosis in the pulmonary vasculature. Assessment should include Doppler leg US imaging and computed tomography pulmonary angiography (CTPA) or ventilation perfusion (V/Q) scanning.

CTPA reveals PE in varying numbers depending on illness severity and access to CTPA scanning. In meta-analyses, where a third of patients underwent CTPA (thus PE prevalence is probably underestimated), estimates of PE were 15% in patients on general wards, and 23% for those in ICU. In studies where patients all underwent CTPA on admission to ICU, the prevalence was higher. For example, in a UK study of 72 patients (half were on extracorporeal membrane oxygenation, ECMO), there were 54 thrombotic complications in 42 patients (58%), including 34 pulmonary arterial (47%), 15 peripheral venous (21%), and 5 (7%) systemic arterial thromboses/end-organ embolic complications. CTPA studies of COVID-associated PE suggest segmental/subsegmental pulmonary arteries are more frequently involved compared to main/lobar arteries. Some cases with severe right ventricular (RV) dysfunction are reported, these may be related to larger volume PE, but RV function is also impacted by multiple factors in COVID-19 pneumonitis including the effects of lung parenchymal disease, gas exchange abnormalities, endothelial dysfunction, and inflammation affecting the lung microcirculation. In addition, invasive positive pressure ventilation, high levels of PEEP and hypercapnia can cause acute right heart dysfunction due to increased transmural intra-alveolar pressure, as previously described in ARDS.

Studies therefore confirm that VTE is especially common in hospital-ised patients, especially in critically unwell patients with COVID-19 pneu-monitis. The rates of VTE exceeds even the usually high levels in critically illness, where risk is already elevated relating to the critical illness, immo-bility, indwelling lines, etc. Therefore, in ICU patients, a pragmatic approach is to perform computed tomography (CT) chest with pulmonary angiography, abdomen, pelvis, leg veins on admission to the ICU. Further to detailed assessment of PE, CT can be useful to assess right heart dimen-sions and proximal pulmonary artery dilatation. Furthermore, transtho-racic echocardiography is very useful in this setting to assess RV function to risk-assess PE (as well as additional cardiac pathology).

Some hospitals have access to dual energy CT (DECT) scanning or similar techniques to assess small vessel perfusion imaging. Abnormalities in microvascular lung perfusion are common at the onset of severe COVID-19 pneumonitis, which may coexist with classical PE ("macrothrombosis") with wedge shaped perfusion abnormalities, or without PE, creating mottling of perfusion (Figure 4). This finding is

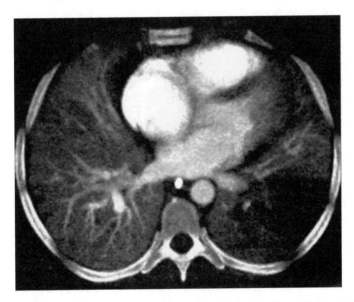

Figure 4. Dual energy CT (DECT) section from patient with severe COVID-19 showing defects in left lower lobe dilated, branching and/or tortuous vessels in the peripheral lung and perfusion defects (Courtesy of Professor Simon Padley, Royal Brompton Hospital).

likely to reflect pulmonary microvascular disease and be a CT sign of immunothrombosis. To support this, microvascular injury is seen in both areas of CT-confirmed parenchymal injury and in areas free of CT-confirmed lung injury using post-mortem studies. However, detailed radiological-pathology studies correlating these observations with post-mortem findings with CT that also combines a DECT component are lacking. The frequently observed microvascular involvement is likely to contribute to the profound respiratory failure seen. Interestingly, the CT signs of microthrombosis on DECT scanning correlate with echocardiographic signs of right ventricular dysfunction more than classical scoring methods of PE burden such as the Qanadli score.

Blood parameters

In addition to imaging, daily monitoring of full blood count, platelet count, prothrombin time (PT), activated partial thromboplastin time (aPTT), fibrinogen, and D-dimer levels should be performed in all patients admitted to hospitals, especially those treated in ICU irrespective of the presence of thrombosis. Daily monitoring allows for any worsening of change/pattern in these parameters which would indicate disease progression and alert clinicians to the requirement for a more aggressive management approach. Moreover, improvement in these markers can be a reassuring indication of recovery and advocate a step down in management.

FBC including platelet count

Assessment of platelet count is essential as it will guide the intensity of anticoagulation and other interventions in patients with thrombosis such as the use of thrombolysis in severe cases of thrombosis. Thrombocytopenia is relatively uncommon in patients with COVID-19 compared to patients with severe disease due to other infections. Patients with severe COVID-19 can present with thrombocytopenia which is often mild (platelet count of $100–150 \times 10^9/L$). Severe thrombocytopenia ($<50 \times 10^9/L$) is related to poor prognosis. A late phase thrombocytopenia, notable 3 weeks following symptom onset has been described but is uncommon. Immune thrombocytopenia associated with COVID-19 has been reported, presenting with an isolated low platelet count.

PT/APTT

PT and APTT can be mildly prolonged in patients with severe disease in keeping with a disseminated intravascular coagulation (DIC)-like state, however prolongation is milder than in classic DIC. These are not contraindications to thromboprophylaxis in patients with COVID-19. In these patients, PT prolongation is often more notable than the APTT, most likely due to an increase in plasma concentration of acute phase reactants; mainly factor VIII and fibrinogen levels.

Additionally, a subset of COVID-19 patients may have a shortened APTT due to similar effects. Shortening of the PT has also been reported in this cohort. A shortened PT in up to 30% of patients with COVID-19 is likely due to increased plasma fibrinogen concentration.

An isolated prolonged APTT can be caused by the presence of a lupus anticoagulant (LA) and has been described in patients with COVID-19. This commonly becomes negative on subsequent retesting. The phenomenon of transient antiphospholipid antibody (aPL)-positivity is recognised in individuals with acute viral infections and does not necessarily represent a diagnosis of antiphospholipid syndrome. It should also be noted that presence of a LA causing artefactual prolongation of the APTT does not indicate an increased bleeding risk unless they are masking an underlying bleeding tendency (will have a bleeding history) or have associated hypoprothrombinemia (will have associated prolonged PT).

As it does not reflect a decreased risk of thromboembolic complications, patients with a LA should receive anticoagulation if indicated. In fact, although the clinical significance of LA in COVID-19 is not fully delineated, LA-positivity may correlate with thrombosis in individuals with COVID-19 and may warrant assessment for more intensive anticoagulation regimens. Also note that APTT prolongation may necessitate using an anti-Xa activity assay to monitor unfractionated heparin, discussed further later.

Fibrinogen

As discussed previously, COVID-19 coagulopathy has been somewhat distinct from the classical ISTH DIC criteria seen in severe sepsis, for example. In COVID-19 an elevated fibrinogen is commonly seen and is a result of enhanced liver production of fibrinogen in response to a systemic inflammatory response. Hypofibrinogenemia (<1 g/L) is less common and in fact a late phenomenon.

D-dimer

D-dimer is a product of cross-linked fibrin and is therefore a sensitive biomarker in this context. D-dimer levels are frequently elevated in patients with COVID-19 and often raised far out of proportion to the degree of abnormalities detected in platelet count, PT, APTT, or fibrinogen. A raised D-dimer can be as a result of both thrombosis and inflammation as it is a non-specific acute phase reactant. Therefore, a normal level of D-dimer may exclude VTE in patients with a low clinical probability, but an elevated D-dimer does not necessarily equate to the presence of VTE. The D-dimer has also proven to have prognostic value with higher levels being associated with more severe clinical outcomes. Data has also demonstrated that those with highly elevated D-dimer levels have an increased risk of thrombosis. D-dimer levels were discussed as having enough significance to stratify COVID-19 thrombotic risk and adjusting anticoagulation intensity; however, this has been questioned given concerns for D-dimer performance in isolation at higher values and the variability with assay methodologies. As such we recommend against using the D-dimer as a sole criterion for mandating decisions regarding investigation and anticoagulation. Instead, levels should be assessed within the overall clinical context due to the lack of conclusive evidence.

When considering the association of high D-dimer concentration and VTE diagnosis, the role of the Wells score as well as D-dimer thresholds are not clear in the setting of COVID-19. No single cut-off value of elevated D-dimer concentration has been agreed upon as a threshold for radiological investigations. The International Society of Thrombosis and Haemostasis considered that a 3–4-fold increase in D-dimer concentration may be significant. One UK study used a cut-off of 2,494 ng/mL for a PE diagnosis using CPTA where sensitivity was 100% (95% CI: 100–100) and specificity of 90.62% (95% CI: 90.5–90.8) for predicting PE. Ideally, we would recommend CTPA and/or limb imaging where practicable, but there may be settings where imaging modalities are unavailable.

In a prospective study of hospitalised patients with COVID-19, the strategy of using D-dimer levels of >1,000 ng/mL did not prove to be useful for risk stratification in asymptomatic patients. Ultimately, clinical judgement must prevail and the threshold for evaluation or diagnosis of DVT and PE should be low, given the high frequency of these events.

In the context of anticoagulation, the REMAP-CAP, ACTIV-4, and ATTACC study groups recently published their combined pooled open-label RCTs of therapeutic LMWH. A treatment benefit was observed in patients with both low (D-dimer <2 times the upper limit of normal per local assay) and high-levels (D-dimer ≥2 times the upper limit of normal per local assay) but the treatment effect was more pronounced in patients with higher levels of D-dimer.

Viscoelastic (VE) assays

Viscoelastic (VE) assays such as Thromboelastography (TEG) and rotational thromboelastometry (ROTEM) are both global haemostatic tests which are performed on whole blood. Using a continuously applied rotational force they assess clot formation, clot strength, and dissolution. The conventional coagulation tests described above do not always fully reflect haemostasis and furthermore are not immediately available for decision making next to the patients. Furthermore, VE assays can reveal coagulopathy, even when this is not detected in routine coagulation tests. COVID-19 patients often harbour abnormalities in coagulation therefore assessing these quickly are paramount to determine a hypocoagulable, hypercoagulable, or abnormal fibrinolytic state. VE assays soon demonstrated that unlike the characteristic DIC picture, COVID-19 coagulopathy progressed more to a hypercoagulable rather than hypocoagulable state. Furthermore, it revealed that alongside increased thrombin generation, fibrin and platelets were also central to clot formation and stability. ROTEM has identified accelerated clot formation and increased clot strength in COVID-19 patients alongside an increased contribution of both platelets and fibrinogen to clot strength. As discussed previously fibrinolysis shutdown was noted, where the absence of lysis at 30 minutes combined with D-dimers levels >2,600 ng/mL was also strongly associated with VTE.

The hypercoagulable profile of COVID-19 has been demonstrated by several studies using VE assays and have generally demonstrated:

- Shortened clot formation time (K): increased fibrin generation
- Increased maximum amplitude (MA): greater clot strength
- Reduced clot lysis at 30 minutes (LY30): with reduced fibrinolysis
- Shortened reaction time (R): early thrombin burst

Although considered "global" tests of coagulation they are poorly sensitive to platelet function disorders amongst many other factors. As with D-dimers, the inter-laboratory and methodology variation is high, and they can be subject to several pre-analytical variables. Although regularly used in trauma, their value in an inflammatory setting such as COVID-19 is yet to be determined and requires more prospective study.

Management

Management of COVID-associated thrombosis can be challenging. It has been demonstrated that hypercoagulability adversely impacts prognosis, however antithrombotic therapy carries with it increased risks of bleeding. Here we discuss safe and appropriate anticoagulation regimens both during admission and on discharge as well as the management of acute thrombosis. Furthermore, we will consider the monitoring of thrombo-prophylaxis and therapeutic anticoagulation as well as the management of patients admitted on existing therapeutic anticoagulants.

Thromboprophylaxis

In the absence of contraindications and careful evaluation of bleeding risk, all hospitalised adults with COVID-19 should receive thrombo-prophylaxis to prevent thrombosis

Hospitalised patients with COVID-19 inherently possess shared pro-thrombotic risk factors with acutely unwell medical patients. These include immobility, advanced age, and the presence of underlying comorbidities. Risk stratification for thrombosis in these patients has remained a point of discussion throughout the pandemic. All patients requiring admission require assessment of their bleeding and thrombotic risk as soon as possible after admission. This should be documented in the patients notes. Although evidence has not demonstrated an increased risk of bleeding with higher doses of anticoagulation, bleeding events remain an adverse consequence of anticoagulant treatment and as such a risk assessment reveals patients at high risk early on in the admission process and prevents harm.

Most UK hospitals integrate a risk assessment tool into their admission process to ensure it is not overlooked. VTE and bleeding risks should be reassessed daily. An individualised assessment of the patient's risk of thrombosis and bleeding is important when deciding on anticoagulation intensity. It should also be noted that in the absence of bleeding, coagulopathy is not a contraindication to heparin unless platelets fall below 30 for prophylaxis or below 50 for therapeutic heparin. Importantly, a change in clinical condition of the patient should prompt an assessment of the risk of VTE, bleeding risk and review of VTE prophylaxis/treatment appropriately.

Optimal intensity and duration of thromboprophylaxis as well as post-discharge prophylaxis have been at the centre of many observational and interventional studies most notably the ATTACC, ACTIV-4a, and REMAP-CAP studies.

REMAP-CAP, ACTIV-4, and ATTACC open label clinical trials span four continents and shared a common goal in establishing any benefit of therapeutic dose anticoagulation over lower dose anticoagulation in moderately ill or critically ill adults requiring hospitalisation for COVID-19. In all three trials, a total of 14 days of heparin was given to patients or until hospital discharge if that was sooner. Instead of thrombosis and bleeding as primary outcomes, these trails opted for mortality primary outcomes and the number of days free from organ support in critical care at day 21.

For patients with moderate disease, the trial was in fact prematurely terminated based on the therapeutic anticoagulation arm demonstrating superiority over standard of care thromboprophylaxis. In this group, prophylactic anticoagulation at therapeutic doses was in fact more associated with improved survival [odds ratio (OR) 1.57 (95% confidence interval 1.14–2.19)]. Furthermore, there were more patients with organ support-free days with therapeutic dosing (80% versus 76%; OR 1.27, 95% CI 1.03–1.58). Other outcomes were not statistically different with therapeutic versus prophylactic dosing. These included: thrombosis (1.1% versus 2.1%), survival to hospital discharge (93% versus 92%; OR 1.21, 95% CI 0.87–1.68), and bleeding (1.9% versus 0.9%; OR 1.80, 95% CI 0.90–3.74).

In patients with severe disease, therapeutic dosing was associated with slightly lower rates of thrombosis (7.2% versus 11.1%) and major thrombosis (6.4% versus 10.4%) compared with prophylactic dosing. Bleeding was also slightly higher with therapeutic dosing but not statistically different (3.8% versus 2.3%; OR 1.48, 95% CI 0.75–3.04).Though not statistically different, there were fewer organ support-free days up to day 21 in the therapeutic dosing group (OR 0.83, 95% CI 0.67–1.03). Survival to hospital discharge was also not statistically different between the two groups (65% versus 63%; OR 0.84, 95% CI: 0.64–1.11). It is important to note however that a high proportion of patients in the prophylactic arm received intermediate dosing which may have impacted results.

The differences in these findings may be due to the population statistics of this data. There is a geographical and ethnic variation between all participants that may have affected results with critically ill patients largely being recruited from the UK and the moderate group mostly USA and South America based. As noted, the "standard dose" arm prophylaxis was left at the discretion of the physician resulting in a variety of both conventional standard and intermediate doses being utilised which may have worked to dilute the effects of full therapeutic dose anticoagulation.

Other studies include the ACTION trial which compared treatment dose anticoagulation using the DOAC (mainly rivaroxaban) for 30 days, with standard prophylactic dose anticoagulant (unfractionated heparin or enoxaparin) in 615 hospitalised patients with predominantly moderate COVID-19. Therapeutic anticoagulation did not improve death or hospitalisation duration. There was no increase in major bleeding but instead, an increase in clinically relevant non-major bleeding with therapeutic anticoagulation compared to standard dose anticoagulant from 2% to 8%.

The INSPIRATION trial was a randomised controlled trial that investigated the effect of intermediate-dose (enoxaparin 1 mg/kg once daily) against standard dose anticoagulation (enoxaparin 40 mg once daily) in 562 ITU patients. There was no difference in the rates of VTE, extracorporeal membrane oxygenation (ECMO) requirement or death between the two groups but increased bleeding was noted in the intermediate dose group.

A summary of the above clinical trials is presented in Table 1.

REMAP-CAP and RECOVERY trials assessed the use of antiplatelet treatment in patients with COVID-19 and showed no benefit.

Antiplatelet Treatment

Given its antithrombotic properties and inexpensive cost, aspirin has been proposed as a treatment for COVID-19. The RECOVERY trial was established as a randomised, controlled, open-label platform trial. A total of 7,351 patients were randomised to aspirin 150 mg once daily and 7,541 patients randomised to standard of care alone. The primary outcome was 28-day mortality. There was no significant difference in the primary endpoint of 28-day mortality (17% aspirin versus 17% standard care). Notably, there was no significant difference in the proportion of patients

Table 1. Summary of management studies in COVID 19-associated thrombosis.

	ICU	Ward	Mixed ward/ICU cohort
Therapeutic anticoagulation	REMAP-CAP, ACTIV-4, and ATTACC**	REMAP-CAP, ACTIV-4, and ATTACC* RAPID**	HEP-COVID* ACTION (rivaroxaban)**
Intermediate dose	INSPIRATION**		
Anti-platelet treatment	REMAP-CAP**	RECOVERY**	

Notes: *Indicates therapeutic dose anticoagulation with heparin is superior to standard dose anticoagulation; **Inferior to standard dose heparin or treatment did not show benefit or cause more harm.

in either arm who progressed to invasive mechanical ventilation or death (21% versus 22%; risk ratio 0.96; 95% CI: 0.90–1.03; $p = 0.23$).

Recommendations

- In stable in-patients managed on general wards and requiring supplemental oxygen, therapeutic low molecular weight heparin (LMWH) should be considered.
- In critically ill patients who require high-flow oxygen, continuous positive airway pressure (CPAP), non-invasive ventilation (NIV) for severe ventilatory failure or invasive ventilation we would *suggest* using prophylactic-intensity over intermediate-intensity or therapeutic-intensity anticoagulation as thromboprophylaxis
- The balance of bleeding risk against thrombotic risk should be assessed in all patients and in patients with risk factors for bleeding, the dose of heparin should be tailored to the individual patient.
- Patients not on supplemental oxygen with an incidental COVID-19 finding, standard thromboprophylaxis dose according to actual body weight and calculated CrCl, antiplatelet treatment is not recommended as prophylaxis in hospitalised patients with COVID-19.

Management of Acute Thrombosis

Patients with COVID-19 with acute thrombosis should be treated in line with other patients with thrombosis taking risk factors for bleeding such as platelet count, renal function and the presence of bleeding already into consideration. Established and validated guidelines should be used in hospitalised patients.

Options include:

- Standard weight-based, renal function-adjusted, therapeutic dose LMWH alone or followed by warfarin (INR target range 2–3).
- UFH/LMWH lead-in therapy with a switch to dabigatran/edoxaban.
- Standard weight-based, renal function-adjusted, therapeutic dose apixaban/rivaroxaban or edoxaban as monotherapy.

Duration of anticoagulation for those with acute thrombosis can vary. The development of VTE in patients with COVID-19-related disease should be considered as a provoked event. Provoking factors include prolonged immobility, a pro-inflammatory, pro-coagulant state, and a damaged endothelium. As such, anticoagulation duration should be at least 3–6 months.

Patients with pulmonary embolism should be followed up in a joint respiratory/haematology clinic to review appropriateness of stopping anticoagulation and review any long-term sequelae of the PE.

Choice of Anticoagulant

Options for pharmacological anticoagulation will depend on local protocols and should be based on disease severity, renal function, platelet count, additional risk factors for bleeding and whether patients need acute intervention or surgery requiring interruption of anticoagulation. Parenteral anticoagulants can offer fewer drug interactions, better absorption, and ease of monitoring compared to oral anticoagulants. Furthermore, they have potential for reversibility in the event of bleeding. Indeed, all classes of anticoagulants can interact with COVID-specific medications such as antibiotics, antivirals, and other investigative trial drugs — particularly via the CYP3A4 pathway. Caution is advised with dexamethasone which is a combined p-glycoprotein and cyp3A4 inducer and all direct oral anticoagulants are p-glycoprotein substrates, while apixaban and rivaroxaban are moderately metabolised by cyp3A4.

Notably, LMWH has been found to have additional anti-inflammatory and anti-complement effects. By neutralising pro-inflammatory proteins LMWH can support the bi-directional relationship between inflammation and thrombosis. Furthermore, subcutaneous heparin may also bind to the

SARS-COV-2 spike protein and block viral attachment thereby reducing viral cell entry.

The use of LMWH may have further advantages due to the lack of routine monitoring compared to intravenous UFH, which also may require unusually high doses in the context caused by possible heparin resistance due to acute phase reactants.

In the inpatient setting we would advise LMWH and UFH. The Rivaroxaban-based anticoagulation strategy discussed above failed to improve outcomes in COVID-19 in the ACTION trial and as such we would advise against the use of DOACs in this setting.

In the discharge setting, DOACs are advantageous over VKA such as warfarin given their lack of need for routine monitoring. They can however be more complicated to reverse in the event of bleeding.

The risk and benefit for each option should be considered on an individual basis. Furthermore, for those at extremes of body weight or with renal impairment, the choice of anticoagulant and dosing should be adjusted according to locally agreed policies and product characteristics.

Monitoring

Monitoring may be required for certain subgroups of patients to assure therapeutic and non-toxic levels: this is largely using heparin anti-Xa level monitoring of LMWH. Monitoring of heparin anti-Xa levels is not required routinely except in the following circumstances:

- Extremes of body weight: underweight patients (<50 kg) or BMI ≥35 Kg/m²; weight >150 kg
- Renal impairment
- Pregnancy
- Bleeding or extension or development of further thrombosis despite standard dose

If the patient is on unfractionated heparin (UFH), we recommend using heparin anti-Xa level monitoring over activated partial thromboplastin time (APTT) as APTT is not reliable in patients with acute inflammation especially with COVID-19 with significantly raised fibrinogen and factor VIII levels.

Management of Patients Already on Anticoagulation on Admission

For those already receiving anticoagulation for a pre-existing condition when admitted to hospital, anticoagulation should be continued unless there has been a change in clinical circumstances resulting in contraindication to its use.

For those on warfarin or a direct oral anticoagulant (DOAC) consider a switch to LMWH if it better facilitates clinical care, or the patient is deteriorating.

In our national multicentre observational study CA-COVID-19, which included 5,883 patients, we assessed the effects of oral anticoagulation prior to admission on 90-day mortality, ICU admission as well as incidence of thrombosis, major bleeding, and multiorgan failure. In multivariate and adjusted propensity score analyses, the only significant association of no anticoagulants prior to admission was increased admission to ICU [HR 1.98 (95% CI 1.37–2.85)]. Importantly, this benefit of oral anticoagulant use was not offset by any increase in bleeding.

Withholding Anticoagulation

Withholding anticoagulation should be considered if:

- A patient is actively bleeding.
- Therapeutic doses may need to be withheld if platelet count is less than $30–50 \times 10^9/L$ or if the fibrinogen is less than 1.0 g/L.
- Thromboprophylaxis should be withheld if the platelet counts are less than $20–30 \times 10^9/L$ or if the fibrinogen is less than 0.5 g/L.

Thrombolysis: Systemic and Catheter-Directed

The British Thoracic Society recommends thrombolysis for patients with massive (high risk) PE, as for non-COVID-19 infected patients. The risk of potential bleeding, however, should not be underestimated. However, catheter-directed approaches have been reported in this cohort applied in severe disease without immediate bleeding complications.

Thrombolysis with tissue plasminogen activator (tPA) is appropriate in COVID in line with usual indications, unless there is a contraindication:

- Limb-threatening DVT
- Massive PE
- Acute stroke
- Acute myocardial infarction (MI)

Consultation with the pulmonary embolism response team (PERT) or stroke team in decision-making is advised, if possible.

Further studies are required to investigate this potential therapeutic approach.

Additional Respiratory Management

Some hospitalised patients with COVID-19 require prolonged periods on supplementary oxygen, and a proportion develop respiratory failure requiring mechanical ventilation. Profound hypoxaemia occurs early on, even before a fall in lung compliance, and likely relates to several factors in the profoundly inflamed lung, including endothelial dysfunction with shunting, early microvascular, macrovascular and lung parenchymal injury, resulting in ventilation perfusion mismatching and disturbed hypoxic pulmonary vasoconstriction.

The decision to admit a patient with COVID-19 to hospital and their management depends on illness severity. When possible, patients with suspected or laboratory-confirmed COVID-19 should undergo initial remote triage. All patients with dyspnoea, oxygen saturations (SpO2) ≤94% on room air (at sea level), concerning symptoms and pre-existing cardiopulmonary disease should be assessed face to face, and those with dyspnoea should be followed closely to assess for worsening respiratory status. National guidelines, for example, those published by the NIH, consider four levels of risk stratification of disease severity. Recommendations are mostly based on moderately strong evidence from randomised trial data, with evidence supporting dexamethasone and remdesivir for those in hospital requiring supplementary oxygen; addition of immune therapies including baricitinib or tocilizumab for patients needing high flow oxygen or non-invasive ventilation (NIV), and dexamethasone plus tocilizumab started within 24 hours of ICU admission for the most severe cases requiring invasive ventilation or ECMO.

In terms of respiratory management, provision of supplemental oxygen and close observation for progression of respiratory failure is key. Some patients need additional non-invasive ventilation, invasive mechanical ventilation, and ECMO. The careful selection of patients for ECMO has led to encouraging outcomes despite long hospital admissions and associated complications. Some cases develop true severe lung fibrosis, with selected patients even, rarely, requiring lung transplantation. The mainstay of treatment is supportive therapy, with additional therapeutic targets including immune therapies as above, secondary bacterial infections and iatrogenic thrombotic complications.

Right ventricular dysfunction is common in severe COVID-19 pneumonitis but does not usually need specific intervention. In some cases of more severe RV dysfunction with end organ dysfunction, specific therapies may be indicated. In patients with PE, thrombolysis is indicated as per BTS guidelines. Thrombolysis has been used as a rescue therapy in patients with multiorgan dysfunction and evidence for microthrombosis on DECT without PE, with early improvement in gas exchange, and no reports of major bleeding, at least in small series, pending prospective studies. Therapies augmenting RV function include vasopressors, inodilators, diuretics, and pulmonary vasodilators, where short-term improvements in oxygenation have been reported, likely related to improved cardiac output. Whether targeting the pulmonary microcirculation with immune modulation, anticoagulation, and endothelial dysfunction might improve lung recovery is as yet unknown.

Follow-Up: Haematological Management

The risk of hospital-associated VTE for medical inpatients is greatest in the first 6 weeks post-discharge. Outside of the COVID era, extended prophylaxis on discharge raised concerns for bleeding risk and post-discharge prophylaxis was largely discouraged. However, conflicting data also support the use of prophylactic LMWH or DOACs in selected populations of high VTE risk with low bleeding risk and in fact reduced the risk of VTE. There is no specific RCT data to guide the optimal duration of thromboprophylaxis in patients recovering from moderate or severe COVID-19. In fact, despite evidence suggesting a higher risk of VTE during hospitalisation in patients with COVID-19 than in patients without COVID-19, reassuringly many observational studies have in fact noted a low incidence of VTE post discharge that is no greater than non-COVID-19 patients.

In the absence of adequate clinical evidence specifically in patients with COVID-19, it is not possible to make specific recommendations about offering routine extended thromboprophylaxis in this cohort. The optimal agent or duration is unclear and more data in this arena is required.

However high-risk patients should be assessed on a case-by case basis and if deemed appropriate with a low bleeding risk, extended thromboprophylaxis may be instituted. High-risk patients may include those with a previous VTE or pregnant patients, for example. Both the choice of agent and duration should also be considered on a case-by-case basis on review of the bleeding and thrombotic risk profile following discussion with the patient.

In the event of a complex case, expert advice can be sought from a haematologist.

Is there a role for follow-up assessment with D-dimer in patients with COVID-19?

The D-dimer has been a useful biomarker of hypercoagulability in COVID-19 hospitalised patients although not reliable in diagnosing thrombosis. In the follow-up period sequential measurement of D-dimer may provide useful information on tailoring the anticoagulant management.

The modified IMPROVE [International Medical Prevention Registry on Venous Thromboembolism VTE) score uses elevated D-dimer (>2 times ULN) to identify patients at an almost three-fold higher risk for VTE in whom there is a significant benefit for extended-duration thromboprophylaxis. This score can be used to guide clinicians with VTE risk mitigation in those who are at low risk of bleeding and with key VTE risk factors such as advanced age, lengthy stay in the ICU, cancer, a prior history of VTE, thrombophilia, severe immobility, an elevated D-dimer (>2 times ULN), and an IMPROVE VTE score of 4 or more. There remains however minimal data in this cohort in this period thus caution should be applied when adjusting anticoagulant strategies based on a single biomarker.

Follow-up: Respiratory

Patients frequently report fatigue and dyspnea following resolution of their acute illness, the so-called "long-COVID" syndrome. Dyspnoea is reported more commonly in survivors of severe illness, for example in 80% of a severe UK post ICU cohort at 6 weeks, and 12% in a mostly severe Chinese cohort at 3 months. Follow up of patients after COVID-19 and those who remain symptomatic following community cases is important as some may have residual or treatable disease. Access to lung function has been limited in many centres due to aerosol generation, but now early lung function and CT studies are emerging. Exercise assessments such as sit to stand tests are useful to assess oxygen desaturation. Formal cardiopulmonary exercise testing may be useful in some patients.

So far, lung function studies indicate that although spirometric indices appear to be generally well preserved, a defect in diffusing capacity (DLco) is common. Reduction in total lung capacity is also reported. These initial findings therefore suggest features of an interstitial/vascular abnormality rather than an airway problem. The low DLCO is associated with severity of illness, pulmonary interstitial changes on CT and oxygen desaturation. Initial studies using cardiopulmonary exercise testing and gas transfer coefficient using nitrous oxide (TLNO) suggest the low gas transfer probably relates to persistent membrane changes rather than due to an isolated reduction in capillary volume. Dysfunctional breathing syndromes are common and can be difficult to manage.

Follow-up lung CT studies from patients with severe disease show that lung changes mostly completely resolve. Those with residual changes mostly show resolving ground glass opacification and interstitial thickening; about a third of patients having fibrotic-like abnormalities, but few have true fibrosis. These changes may not be detected on chest radiography. Some patients have residual minor pulmonary thromboembolic disease seen on CTPA and/or VQ scanning. Comprehensive follow-up studies of patients following major COVID-19-associated acute PE (macrothrombosis) and microthrombosis are however awaited. Additional imaging modalities are available in some centres including dual energy lung CT and MR lung to image small vessels. V/Q scanning is also useful and more commonly available. Comparator studies between these imaging techniques in this setting are awaited. Despite the prevalence of RV dysfunction in patients with severe COVID-19 pneumonitis, with or without PE, pulmonary hypertension fortunately does not appear to be a common long-term problem, except in rare patients with severe lung fibrosis, i.e., group 3 pulmonary hypertension.

In terms of physiological recovery, symptoms and lung function deficits appear to improve over time in most patients. The trajectory and extent of recovery is yet to be reported however, and some patients do have a slower recovery profile with some remaining symptomatic. From the randomised study data available so far, a 6-week rehabilitation exercise program had a positive effect on walking distance and recovery of lung function, most notably DLCO. The potential impact of anticoagulant, antiplatelet and immune therapeutic agents on long term respiratory outcomes remains to be seen.

Bearing in mind the limited current available evidence, a reasonable follow up approach is as follows:

- Consider prolonged thromboprophylaxis for hospitalised patients recovering from moderate to severe COVID-19, using an individualised approach.
- Following confirmed VTE, given the provoked nature of COVID-19, uncomplicated cases should receive 3–6 months anticoagulation.
- Patients following critical illness due to COVID-19 and those with breathlessness should be assessed to understand the aetiology of symptoms and for residual cardiopulmonary disease.
- Multimodal respiratory assessment includes exercise assessment, CXR, full lung function including gas transfer, cardiac biomarkers, ECG, and echocardiography. As chest radiography may miss parenchymal and pulmonary vascular disease, CT and V/Q scanning are useful, especially in patients with abnormal lung function.
- Cardiopulmonary exercise testing may be useful in selected cases.
- Pulmonary rehabilitation should be encouraged in most cases.

Conclusion

Thrombosis and coagulopathy are frequent complications in patients with COVID-19. A better understanding of these pathophysiological mechanisms is essential for the development of safe and efficient treatment strategies. There has been extraordinary development of several research lines evaluating antithrombotic therapies at a worldwide level. Based on current clinical trial data, in stable in-patients managed on general wards who require supplemental oxygen, therapeutic LMWH should be considered. In critically ill patients who require high-flow oxygen, CPAP, NIV for severe ventilatory failure or invasive ventilation we would *suggest* using prophylactic-intensity over intermediate-intensity or therapeutic-intensity anticoagulation as thromboprophylaxis. The balance between bleeding and thrombotic risk should be assessed in all patients and in patients with risk factors for bleeding, the dose of heparin should be tailored to the individual patient. There is no role for antiplatelet treatment as prophylaxis in hospitalised patients with COVID-19. Patients with acute thrombosis should be treated in line with other patients presenting with acute thrombosis. The choice of anticoagulation should depend on the perceived risk of bleeding, platelet count, COVID-19 disease severity and renal function. Patients with thrombosis, especially those who have developed PE, should be reviewed and assessed for the presence of complications in a joint PE clinic with a haematologist and a respiratory physician. The duration of anticoagulation should be a minimum of 3–6 months and requirement for longer duration should be decided in the follow up clinic. At present, there is no evidence to support the use and duration of routine thromboprophylaxis at discharge from hospital. An individuated approach to each patient should be adopted when deciding on thromboprophylaxis at discharge with input from the haematology team.

Acknowledgement

We would like to thank Professor Simon Padley, consultant radiologist, Royal Brompton Hospital for providing the DECT image.

Bibliography

Akoluk, A., Mazahir, U., Douedi, S. *et al.* (2020). Pulmonary embolism in COVID-19 treated with VA-ECLS and catheter tPA, *Clinical Medicine Insights: Circulatory, Respiratory and Pulmonary Medicine*, 14, pp. 1179548420957451.

Arachchillage, D.J., Rajakaruna, I., Odho, Z. *et al.* (2021). Clinical outcomes and the impact of prior oral anticoagulant use in patients with coronavirus disease 2019 admitted to hospitals in the UK — A multicentre observational study, *British Journal of Haematology*, 196, pp. 79–94.

Arachchillage, D.J., Stacey, A., Akor, F., Scotz, M., and Laffan, M. (2020). Thrombolysis restores perfusion in COVID-19 hypoxia, *British Journal of Haematology*, 190(5), pp. e270–e274.

ATTACC Investigators, ACTIV-4a Investigators, REMAP-CAP Investigators *et al.* (2021). Therapeutic anticoagulation with heparin in noncritically ill patients with COVID-19, *The New England Journal of Medicine*, 385(9), pp. 790–802.

Gao, Y., Chen, R., Geng, Q., Mo, X., Zhan, C., Jian, W. *et al.* (2021). Cardiopulmonary exercise testing might be helpful for interpretation of impaired pulmonary function in recovered COVID-19 patients, *European Respiratory Journal*, 57, pp. 2004265.

INSPIRATION Investigators, Sadeghipour, P., Talasaz, A.H. *et al.* (2021). Effect of intermediate-dose vs standard-dose prophylactic anticoagulation on thrombotic events, extracorporeal membrane oxygenation treatment, or mortality among patients with COVID-19 admitted to the intensive care unit: The INSPIRATION randomized clinical trial, *JAMA*, 325(16), pp. 1620–1630.

John Wort, S., Arachchillage, D.J., McCabe, C., and Price, L.C. (2020). Covid-19 pneumonia and pulmonary vascular disease: A UK Centre perspective, *Respiratory Medicine and Research*, 78, pp. 100781.

Kianzad, A., Meijboom, L.J., Nossent, E.J. *et al.* (2021). COVID-19: Histopathological correlates of imaging patterns on chest computed tomography, *Respirology*, 26(9), pp. 869–877.

Liu, K., Zhang, W., Yang, Y., Zhang, J., Li, Y., and Chen, Y. (2020). Respiratory rehabilitation in elderly patients with COVID-19: A randomized controlled study, *Complementary Therapies in Clinical Practice*, 39, pp. 101166.

Patel, B.V., Arachchillage, D.J., Ridge, C.A. *et al.* (2020). Pulmonary angiopathy in severe COVID-19: Physiologic, imaging, and hematologic observations, *American Journal of Respiratory and Critical Care Medicine*, 202(5), pp. 690–699.

Price, L.C., Ridge, C., and Wells, A.U. (July 2021). Pulmonary vascular involvement in COVID-19 pneumonitis: Is this the first and final insult? *Respirology*, 26(9), pp. 832–834.

Taha, M. and Samavati, L. (2021). Antiphospholipid antibodies in COVID-19: A meta-analysis and systematic review, *RMD Open*, 7(2), pp. e001580.

Index

CPSIA information can be obtained
at www.ICGtesting.com
Printed in the USA
LVHW082024010323
740608LV00002B/17